Psychiatric and Mental Health Nursing: The Field of Knowledge

Edited by

Stephen Tilley

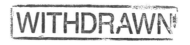
Blackwell
Science

© 2005 by Blackwell Science Ltd
a Blackwell Publishing company

Editorial offices:
Blackwell Science Ltd, 9600 Garsington Road, Oxford OX4 2DQ, UK
   Tel: +44 (0) 1865 776868
Blackwell Publishing Inc., 350 Main Street, Malden, MA 02148-5020, USA
   Tel: +1 781 388 8250
Blackwell Science Asia Pty Ltd, 550 Swanston Street, Carlton, Victoria 3053, Australia
   Tel: +61 (0)3 8359 1011

First published 2005

Library of Congress Cataloging-in-Publication Data
Psychiatric and mental health nursing : the field of knowledge / edited by Stephen Tilley.
   p. ; cm.
Includes bibliographical references and index.
ISBN 0-632-05845-5 (pbk. : alk. paper)
1. Psychiatric nursing–Great Britain.   2. Psychiatric nursing–Study and teaching–Great
Britain.   3. Psychiatric nursing–Philosophy.
[DNLM: 1. Psychiatric Nursing–Great Britain.   2. Education, Nursing–Great Britain.
3. Mental Disorders–nursing–Great Britain.   4. Nursing Theory–Great Britain.
WY 160 P9712 2004]   I. Tilley, Stephen.

RC440.P7297 2004
616.89′0231–dc22

                                                    2004009497

ISBN 0-632-05845-5

A catalogue record for this title is available from the British Library

Set in 10/12.5pt Palatino
by Graphicraft Limited, Hong Kong
Printed and bound in India
by Replika Press Pvt. Ltd, Kundli

The publisher's policy is to use permanent paper from mills that operate a sustainable
forestry policy, and which has been manufactured from pulp processed using acid-free and
elementary chlorine-free practices. Furthermore, the publisher ensures that the text paper
and cover board used have met acceptable environmental accreditation standards.

For further information on Blackwell Publishing, visit our website:
www.blackwellnursing.com

Contents

This book is dedicated to

Annie Altschul 1919–2001

who brought, gave, and left so much to the field

'The field cannot well be seen from within the field.'

Ralph Waldo Emerson.

Foreword

This book was designed to give a picture of the field of knowledge of UK Psychiatric and Mental Health Nursing. The strategy for doing this is described in the Introduction. The core of the book is a set of seven accounts by UK authors of nursing knowledge as institutionalised in their academic institutions. In some of these chapters authors also explore tensions between experiential and professional knowledge of mental illness. There is then a collective reflection on the field, made up of each author's response to the papers by all the other authors. Then, to widen the reflexive arc all these documents were read by international respondents, who commented on the UK authors' text in light of their own sense of the field in their own countries. Finally, a sociologist, familiar with issues of mental health nursing, read all this material and provided an interpretation of some salient features of the accounts from a sociology of knowledge perspective.

The reader will, therefore get most from reading the book in its entirety and in sequence. However, readers wanting to read selectively will learn about different perspectives on mental health nursing practice, education and research by reading individual chapters in Section 2; those interested in brief, well-informed accounts of mental health nursing issues in selected countries outwith the UK might like to start with Section 3. Readers from disciplines outwith nursing, particularly sociology and social policy, might find it useful to read Chapter 12 first, as a view of the field refracted through a sociological lens.

The chapters and commentaries are written in varying styles, and with varying degrees of reflexivity. The book will be of interest to those psychiatric and mental health nurses who, through individual and collective efforts, construct the field in practice, education and research, and whose experiences cause them to reflect on their relations with their institutions and on the repertoire of knowledges they must master to be effective professionals.

Stephen Tilley
Edinburgh 2004

Acknowledgements

This book is the product of sustained collaborative effort over a long time. I am first of all grateful to all the contributing authors, who entered into a covenant beyond the usual contract of publishing commitments, and stayed faithful to the project on which we embarked. I thank Desmond Ryan for his generosity of mind and spirit, without which I could not have completed my elements of the collective task. The metaphoric extension with which the book concludes I owe to him. Blackwell Publishing 'trusted the process' enabling outcome: I thank them on behalf of all contributors.

Stephen Tilley
Edinburgh 2004

Contributors

Alexander McMurdo Carson, RN, RNT, Dip Nurs (London), MSc, PhD
Reader in Nursing Studies, Faculty of Medical Education and Health, North-East Wales Institute of Higher Education, Wrexham, Wales

Mary Chambers, BEd (Hons), DPhil, RGN, RMN, DN (London), RNT
Professor of Mental Health Nursing and Chief Nurse, Kingston University/St George's Medical School and Southwest London Mental Health NHS Trust, London, England

Kathryn Church, BA (Hons), MA (Psych), PhD
Research Associate, Ryerson-RBC Institute for Disability Studies Research and Education, Adjunct Professor, School of Disability Studies, Ryerson University, Toronto, Ontario, Canada

Susanne Forrest, MPhil, Dip CNE, PG Cert Education, RGN, RMN
Senior Lecturer, School of Community Health, Napier University, Edinburgh, Scotland

Vicky Franks, TQAP, MSc, Dip Ned, Dip Psych, RNT, RGN
Vice-Dean and Senior Lecturer in Nurse Education and Consultancy, Tavistock and Portman NHS Trust; Principal Lecturer, School of Health and Social Sciences, Middlesex University, London, England

Ruth Gallop, RN, BSc N, MSc N, PhD
Professor Emeritus, Faculty of Nursing, University of Toronto, Toronto, Canada

David Glenister, BS, MSc, PGCEA, RMN
Lecturer in Nursing, University of Hull, Hull, England

Kevin Gournay, CBE, FRCPsych (Hon), FMedSci, PhD C Psychol, FRCN
Professor, Health Services Research Department, Institute of Psychiatry, London, England

Peter Griffiths, BSc (Hons), SRN, RMN, Cassel Cert
Senior Lecturer in Child and Family Mental Health Nursing/Child and Family Department, The Tavistock Clinic; Principal Lecturer, Middlesex University, London, England

Mike Hazelton, RN, BA, MA, PhD, FANZCMHN
Professor of Mental Health Nursing, The University of Newcastle and Hunter Mental Health, Newcastle, New South Wales, Australia

Madeleine Heron, MPhil (Hons), BSc, BA
Consumer Advisor, University of Auckland, Auckland, New Zealand

Carol E. Kelly, BA (Hons), PG Dip Peace Studies, MA Peace Studies, AIST(LS)
User Consultant; Occasional Lecturer, University of Ulster, Coleraine, and University of Ulster, Magee; Founder member, Unlimited Survivors, Portstewart, Northern Ireland

Hugh Masters, MPhil, PG Cert T&L HE, RMN
Senior Lecturer, School of Community Health, Napier University, Edinburgh, Scotland

Ian Norman, BA, MSc, PhD, RMN, RGN, RNMH, CQSW
Professor of Nursing and Inter-disciplinary Care, Florence Nightingale School of Nursing and Midwifery, King's College London, London, England

Anthony J. O'Brien, RGN, RPN, BA, M Phil (Hons)
Senior Lecturer, Mental Health Nursing, Division of Psychiatry, University of Auckland, Auckland, New Zealand

Tessa Parkes, BSc (Hons), PhD, PGCE, RMN
Senior Lecturer in Health and Social Care, School of Applied Social Science, University of Brighton, Brighton, England

Desmond P. Ryan, MA, DPhil, Dip Soc Admin
Senior Research Fellow, 'Spirited Scotland' Project, Nursing Studies, School of Health in Social Science, University of Edinburgh, Edinburgh, Scotland

Susanne Schoppmann, Dr rer med
Research Fellow and Psychiatric Nurse, Institute of Nursing Science, University of Witten/Herdecke, Nordrhein Westfalen, Germany

Shirley Smoyak, PhD, FAAN
Editor of *Journal of Psychosocial Nursing and Mental Health Services*; Professor, Bloustein School of Planning and Public Policy, Rutgers, The State University of New Jersey, New Brunswick, New Jersey, USA

Stephen Tilley, PhD, BA, RMN, Cert Behavioural Psychotherapy (JBCNS Course 650)
Senior Lecturer, Nursing Studies, School of Health in Social Science, University of Edinburgh, Edinburgh, Scotland

Section 1

Background and Stance on the Problem of
Knowledge in the Field

Chapter 1

Introduction

Stephen Tilley and Desmond Ryan

This book is a study in (and of) the field of knowledge of psychiatric and mental health nursing (PMHNing)[1]. It documents, and is a document of, a collaborative inquiry into the institutionalisation of knowledge in the field, with particular reference to UK higher education. In this Introduction we have three aims: to set out the purpose, topic and focus of the book; to explain what the authors were invited to do, and how they responded to that invitation; and to describe the sociology of knowledge model which informed Ryan's development of a framework for later analysis. The key to understanding the interconnection of these aims is to see them all as making clear how the book was originally conceived and theorised.

The idea for a book on the field of knowledge developed from work on *The Mental Health Nurse: Views of Practice and Education* (Tilley 1997). There, Tilley asked various contributors to convey their views of PMHNing practice and education. The paradigm in the earlier book was knowledge as plurivocal conversation, situated metaphorically in the contemporary agora; in short, as rhetorical, with each contributor seeking to persuade the audience to see the good of (and perhaps follow) his or her practice. While some of the contributors set their versions of practice and knowledge in an institutional context, e.g. admission ward or therapeutic community, there was no remit for self-conscious reference to the institution and institutionalisation of knowledge. By contrast, contributors to the present volume were asked to exercise precisely such institutional reflexivity. Why? We will outline three reasons.

First, by the mid/late 1990s the image of the field had shifted from site of conversation to contested territory. The field had become a site of challenge and counter-challenge over knowledge claims. As the politics of knowledge became

---

[1] 'Psychiatric and mental health nursing' is the term encompassing what are sometimes distinct identities, that of the mental health nurse and the psychiatric nurse (the latter formerly known as 'mental nurse'). See Altschul (1997) on use of these terms. I did not prescribe to authors which term to use, and authors have used whichever term(s) they saw fit. In various places authors remark on the significance of the term they or others have used. In this text PMHN is used as an abbreviation for psychiatric and mental health nurse. In places PMHNing is used as an abbreviation for psychiatric and mental health nursing.

more explicit, the institutional positions from which those writing about the field spoke became more important. This was set in the context of changing institutionalisation of nursing knowledge following the wholesale move of British nursing into higher education in 1992[2]. With this mass move into the academy, issues of knowledge production and dissemination became more important, and individuals' career prospects more closely tied to those of their academic departments and universities (and the Research Assessment Exercise, see below).

Second, along with the new audiences of academic teachers and researchers, and undergraduate and postgraduate PMHNing students, new journals appeared. In particular, the *Journal of Psychiatric and Mental Health Nursing* provided a forum for 'hot' debate on questions such as: Is PMHNing fundamentally concerned with care, with control, or with the tension between these? Is care to be construed as science-based? According to what knowledge paradigm – nomothetic or idiographic, quantitative or qualitative, RCT gold standard or narrative? Is there something unique about knowledge and practice of care in PMHNing? So hot were the debates about knowledge, so polarised and polarising the positions adopted, that Tilley characterised them as 'care wars' (Tilley 1997). The potential for dialogic or plurivocal knowledge development was clear but (Tilley thought) not fully realised.

A notable aspect of both potential and limitation was the personalisation of the debates and arguments. In particular, two figures were seen as articulating contrasting and (apparently) conflicting versions of PMHNing: Kevin Gournay (Section of Psychiatric Nursing, Institute of Psychiatry) and Phil Barker (University of Newcastle-upon-Tyne). These men appeared as 'champions' locked in battle, their moves in argument watched, cheered or challenged by respective 'camps' of supporting academics and practitioners. We will not try to characterise their arguments – some of the texts in this book give a sense of that – but instead note that in the field at that time arguments were addressed and heard as disputes between persons in institutional contexts. Institutional contexts were made relevant, by those in both 'camps', in making and in challenging claims (Gournay 1995, 1997; Barker & Reynolds 1996; Rolfe 1996; Lego 1997; Parsons 1997; Rolfe 1997).

The third aspect relevant to institutional reflexivity is the appeals made, in the course of arguments, to benefit (or cost) to service users: Gournay asserting that users want the most effective interventions appropriately delivered; Barker that the professional has to 'get personal' (Barker 1991) in working with users. These (textually-constructed) positions should be seen in the context of three policy imperatives of that period, all central to the 'modernisation' of the National Health Service. The first was the drive towards evidence-based health care (and

---

[2] Until then, most nurses were trained in 'Colleges of Nursing' linked to hospitals. They followed courses of study interspersed with periods of rostered, paid service, leading to registration. With 'Project 2000', nurse teachers and their students were brought into higher education institutions, the students mostly pursuing pre-graduate diploma courses in nursing with linked registration. Since the 1960s a minority of students have taken undergraduate degree courses in universities, with linked registration. The number of degree courses leading to registration is increasing.

evidence-based practice, services, education . . .); the second was the drive to make the patient the central focus of health service planning and delivery. Both were relevant to debates about the requisite knowledge base for practice, e.g. about whether that knowledge base was uni-disciplinary or multi-disciplinary, and the value and place of professional and patient (user, consumer) knowledges.[3]

These three aspects were closely interrelated, as two examples indicate. Consider first the attention given to the 'Thorn Initiative' programme of courses (initially at the Institute of Psychiatry and at the University of Manchester) providing multi-disciplinary training in psychosocial interventions (PSI). These university-based courses were promoted on the basis of appeals to the evidence base for the effectiveness both of PSIs and of the training itself. These claims for legitimation were articulated in the context of challenges and counter-challenges about their appropriate place in PMHNing practice and education (Gournay 1997; Rolfe 1997). These were, in effect, challenges about the institutionalisation of knowledge. They were critiqued, by Thorn Project proponents, of nurse educational courses purportedly endorsing 'nursing theories' lacking empirical validation.

The challenge was fundamentally about what is to 'count as knowledge' (Berger & Luckmann 1971; Doyle McCarthy 1996). This challenge was even clearer in a second example: the Research Assessment Exercise (RAE) of 2001.[4] Questions of whether and how mental health nursing research would be considered, who would 'count' the knowledge and what would 'count' as knowledge were more vigorously debated as the Exercise approached (Gournay & Ritter 1998; Rolfe 1998; Collectively 2001). Given the role of the RAE in determining a significant element of funding to institutions, for future knowledge production, linkages among the three issues noted above were more evident and more evidently significant. What persons, from which higher education institutions, would evaluate knowledge claims, and on what basis; the power of peer-reviewed journals in mediating research output; and the role of service users in different paradigms of knowledge production: these were all key themes in the politics of knowledge from 1996–2001.

Thus, drawing again on the metaphor of nurse-writers as rhetoricians, we can contrast their position from the mid/late 1990s with that before. They were speaking and writing in a new 'agora'. We can see the traditional elements of the rhetorician's art – *ethos* (the speaker/writer's character), *pathos* (relationship to the audience) and *logos* (the form and content of arguments) (Weaver, cited in Szasz 1979; Tilley 1997) – all changed, in ways difficult to read, in the changing field/'agora'. Essaying a view of this changed context required a different methodology from that in *The Mental Health Nurse*; collective/collaborative argument

---

[3] All these imperatives are expressed in the key document *The New NHS* (Department of Health 1997).
[4] The Research Assessment Exercise is a UK-wide occasional (originally quadrennial) peer-review exercise intended to assess the quality of research done in higher education institutions. Institutions submit research to peer panels based on disciplines or subjects. Nursing research has been submitted mainly to nursing panels but has sometimes been submitted as part of multi-disciplinary entries (see Chapter 2). This is a key issue in the construction of knowledge in the field.

about the field of knowledge of PMHNing, conducted through an appropriately designed text. We turn now to discuss the methodology.

Methodology of the book – architecture of the text

The premiss of this book is that the field in which psychiatric/mental health nurses work lies at the intersection of a set of institutional forces which are as powerful as they are opaque. These forces shape what PMHNs do, write, read, learn, think, perceive, value. Tilley aimed to organise an account of the field that would reveal how it is situated in its academic and professional contexts, and how these contexts condition mental health nursing work. The book would show how those within the field, including users, professionals and policy makers, constitute interest groups, each of which tries to shape the field to its own advantage and contests with others in trying to direct work, education and policy.

The metaphors that informed planning and development of the book (and provided a reference point to which Tilley returns in drawing conclusions) are devices for imagining and writing towards something not clearly known or formulated, 'think withs', to borrow Hodgkin's (1997) phrase. The duo-metaphor guiding development of the book is that of UK psychiatric and mental health nursing as a *field* in which various figures, each in a *tower*, survey the field about them and each other in the field. The towers are the institutions in which these scholars work, in which they represent, in their teaching and their research, the knowledge needed for practice as PMHNs. Each appears as one working to create and sustain his or her variety of knowledge, each variety as distinctive as a medieval ducal crest or flag. While the features of some 'flags' are well known, others are not.

The UK authors of Chapters 2–8 were seen as working in towers, from which they could survey the field. They were asked to write from within their institutions, about how knowledge was institutionalised therein: to turn their gaze inwards in order to see and then convey the field of mental health nursing as that was the subject of knowledge production and communication in their particular institutional contexts. *How* they were to do that Tilley did not specify closely, wanting each to find the form as well as content best suited to that task – as they saw it. (Tilley will return in the Conclusion to consider whether this approach was the best to have taken.)

The use of these metaphors, and the relatively free rein regarding form and content, shaped the process of this collaborative inquiry into British psychiatric/mental health nursing, informed by a sociology of knowledge perspective. The collaborative inquiry proceeded in three 'rounds', of concentrically expanding reflexivity.

Chapters 2–8 (Section 2) constitute the '*first round*'. Each of Chapters 2–8 should be read as addressed in the first instance to the writers of other chapters in that section and then to a set of international commentators. This is because the writers knew that in the 'second round', when Chapters 2–8 were finished, they would read the chapters written by other authors in that section, and comment on the field as they now saw it, in the light of others' views. For this reason, Chapters 2–8 can be read both as stand-alone views of the field as a bit of social reality 'produced and communicated' in and by the authors and colleagues in their settings, and as first moves in further communication about the field.

The remit given to the authors of those chapters was to give reflexive accounts of their own institutions (as teachers, scholars, researchers, or user variant of these). Five of the chapters were written on the basis of the authors' work in various academic institutions: some 'older' (pre-1992) and some newer (post-1992) universities; some in universities that had offered courses and research degrees for 40 years, others in former (training) Schools of Nursing now incorporated into universities; some with international reputations, others less well known. The authors of Chapters 2–6 thus were asked to consider how PMHNing knowledge was institutionalised in their academic settings, to indicate distinguishing aspects of knowledge of PMHNing in their settings, and the role they saw their institution playing in the field of knowledge. They were also asked to consider themselves in relation to their own institution – how they as knowledge producers were situated. Chapter 2 by Prof Kevin Gournay gives a clear picture of the Section of Psychiatric Nursing's contribution to multi-disciplinary research in the Institute of Psychiatry. The Institute is one of the main UK centres of postgraduate education and research for various disciplines involved in mental health work. Chapter 3, by Tilley, provides an account of what he calls the 'fragile' tradition of psychiatric and mental health nursing research and education at the University of Edinburgh, which pioneered development of academic nursing in the UK. In Chapter 4, Peter Griffiths and Vicky Franks convey in rich detail the practice-base and knowledge-base of psychodynamic and systemic psychotherapies at the Cassel Hospital and the Tavistock Institute in London, and nurses' roles in bridging those institutions and the Middlesex University. In Chapter 5, Alex Carson, a general nurse academic at the North East Wales Institute (part of the University of Wales), uses the method of self-reflection to consider critically the principled basis of the curriculum devised and taught by his mental health colleagues. In Chapter 6, Susanne Forrest and Hugh Masters, of Napier University, Edinburgh, describe their research on what users and carers valued in mental health nurses, and the process by which the authors then involved users in teaching and evaluation of students. The co-authors of Chapter 7 (Mary Chambers, David Glenister, Carol Kelly and Tessa Parkes) constructed their account on the basis of their experience of the boundaries of experiential knowledge of mental illness and formal knowledge in academic institutions. Ian Norman, the author of Chapter 8, was asked to contribute reflections on a study funded by the English National Board of Nursing, Midwifery and Health Visiting, in which he and co-researchers developed 'models' of mental health nursing, 'ideal types' of working knowledges in the field.

Emerson's maxim (Emerson 1841) that 'the field cannot well be seen from within the field' informed the 'second round' of the book's construction. The field as a social field could better be seen or imagined if all saw the field from each other's perspective. Chapter 9 contains the products of the second 'round'. Here, the authors of Chapters 2–8 were asked to read all the other chapters from that set, and write reflective commentaries conveying their perceptions of the field in the light of that reading. This chapter is doubly reflexive: each sees the field from within the field in the light of the others' views; each is asked to see perspectively.

Chapter 10 comprises the third 'round', providing international perspectives on the state of knowledge of PMHNing in Britain. Here, scholars from a range of countries, knowledgeable about the field of PMHNing, comment on Chapters 2–9, reflexively constructing their responses by reference to the knowledge and practice base in their own national, cultural and institutional contexts. They are Ruth Gallop (University of Toronto), Mike Hazelton (University of Newcastle and Hunter Mental Health, Australia), Anthony O'Brien and Madeleine Heron (University of Auckland), Susanne Schoppmann (University of Witten-Herdige) and Shirley Smoyak (Rutgers University). Kathryn Church (Ryerson University, Toronto), a sociologist, contributed on the basis of her experience of work at the boundaries of academic and service users/survivors' knowledge, as a community researcher ally of the Toronto's psychiatric survivors community.

Desmond Ryan, a sociologist familiar with UK mental health nursing literature, conveys in Chapter 11 his view of the field based on reading Chapters 2–10. Chapter 12, the Conclusion, returns to the metaphors that guided construction of the book, and to the sociology of knowledge matrix.

The whole field, and nothing but the field?

Tilley's intentions in designing the book in this way were two-fold. On the one hand, writers were conceived of as people committed to versions of psychiatric and mental health nursing, looking over the ramparts of their institutions at the other figures and institutions in the field. The book was intended to give them scope to convey their views in forms and tones that would allow the battle for the soul of the profession to come alive. On the other hand, the book was intended to provide a space for a more distanced, less over-committed view of the field, by the above figures, by scholars from other countries and cultures and by more sociologically-situated perceivers.

Those involved in building professional identities are personally and professionally involved in their work, and bring these commitments into their academic work. The book was intended to provide a lesson in how the professional field conducts its business in academic terms, reflecting major tensions and commitments in the field as construed by participants, and constituting a vehicle for development and expression, through the text as a *whole*, of the academic virtues of reflective, principled argument.

The aim is clearly to give *a* picture of the field, not *the* picture of the field. In different chapters the reader will find some authors questioning the adequacy of the book's scope, and even whether a field is clearly identified. Even granting that the focus is on academic institutions, one can ask why the particular institutions and authors were chosen for inclusion. The selection was based on Tilley's perception that the authors chosen were well placed and able to articulate a view from their respective institutions, and that the institutions were sufficiently varied in size, history and profile to reflect at least in part the variety of the field.

It is appropriate to note those who were asked to contribute but did not. Phil Barker, then Professor of Psychiatric Nursing Practice at the University of Newcastle-upon-Tyne, considered doing a chapter but declined as he thought this might perpetuate the personalised debate which had gone on too long, and as he and colleagues were prioritising work for the Research Assessment Exercise. Len Bowers, then Reader, now Professor of Mental Health Nursing at City University, was asked to contribute, partly in light of his role in setting up and moderating the internet-based Psychiatric Nursing List, an important site of debate at that time; but also declined due to pressure of other work. I asked Professor Charles Brooker, then at the University of Manchester, to do a chapter with colleagues as that institution was a prominent centre of research and training, but he declined when he moved to another institution.

The sociology of knowledge model adopted in this book

'The field of knowledge' might suggest a two- or three-dimensional, static construct. The guiding metaphor, described above, should highlight to the reader that this is not the case here. The field of PMHNing is better understood diachronically, as changing and developing over time.

Ryan devised a framework which we thought might be helpful to the contributors in writing their chapters, and to ourselves in interpreting the various authors' contributions. Let there be[5] two dimensions (see Fig. 1.1). Crossing them produces a four-cell table, with the following as occupant of each cell (see Fig. 1.2): institution, discipline, school/tradition, influence. The competitive dynamic of professional knowledge in the liberal democracies is to move round the circle from bottom left to bottom right. The ambitious holder of powerful

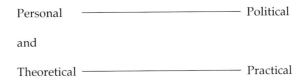

Fig. 1.1   The dimensions of academic-professional knowledge.

---

[5] 'Let there be' is a version of what Burke calls 'entitlement' – bestowing a name and, in doing so, bringing something into being. Any term thus brought into being directs attention to one thing rather than another, and generates a 'terministic screen' (Blankenship 1989).

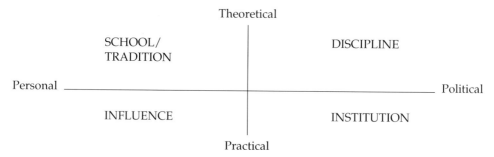

Fig. 1.2   Academic-professional knowledge as a process of power.

knowledge (knowledge that has social consequences) is a powerful knower in each cell, but the form taken by that powerful knowledge is different.

The circle is a series of transitions: on impersonality, on scale and on power. At each transition the personal influence of an individual gets harder to discern, although those centrally involved in the process of the field's knowledge-system are able to map it in detail. Outsiders and low-level insiders may see the workings of *institutions* as impersonal and ideal; insiders and participants experience them as personalised and politicised (Burns 1969). They also appreciate that they are the topmost level of an articulated system of knowledge which stretches from the individual scholar in his/her garret to policies that determine mental health outcomes for thousands.

What were our working definitions of institution, discipline, tradition, and influence?

Institution

Institutions are politico-economic structures which publicly hold knowledge which is interest-bearing, consensually validated, usable. This knowledge is taken from disciplines and traditions, though filtered through a mesh of political judgements as to practicability, congruence with political interests, etc. Modal institutions of this knowledge-bearing kind are:

- The 'professional body'
- The national standards agency
- Departments/courses in higher education
- The clinical system of the healthcare delivery service/agencies.

As political-practical, the institutions control practice, allocate resources (including non-material, e.g. recognition), seal legitimacy, promote leaders, reward teams and launch agendas for change. All of these aspects variably impact on/derive from the discipline sector. When the political system changes, knowledge in institutions becomes an open frontier, an openness that can also affect the disciplinary field.

The history of knowledge in institutions is a succession of authoritative holdings of knowledge-for-use (syllabuses, Schemes of Training, research paradigms and paradigmatic texts, letters of guidance).

Discipline

A discipline is a virtual structure of knowledge in public and competitive (through criticism, whether public or hidden, e.g. 'peer review') process. A discipline is visible in:

- books, journals and professional magazines
- research in progress
- conferences and meetings
- teaching and supervision.

All disciplines are subject to the ideological and values authority of the ideal-typical university, which has overall power to shape what is accepted as disciplinary knowledge.

Disciplinary knowledge is:

- universal
- public (i.e. published)
- textual
- conventional
- open to critique.

The history of a discipline is the history of claims for findings and critiques of claims, of knowledge in good or less good standing with disciplinary members, of guiding questions and controlling paradigms, of the moving frontier of interest and discovery, of argument and debate.

Tradition

A professional tradition is people-knowing-together, in real or virtual personal relationship, synchronically or historically. Knowledge in a tradition or school (a school is a tradition without an ancestor generation) is handled with explicit reference to its provenance from respected individuals with whom the handlers seek to identify. Traditions can evolve in a historical way or be constructed with a degree of artificiality (e.g. 'new' nursing cultures tracing their links to Florence Nightingale).

Unlike the universal, textual and criticisable knowledge of the discipline, the knowledge of the tradition is often esoteric, narrational and related to membership of values-based social groups. Traditions may well handle disciplinary knowledge in the appropriate way, while giving it a values spin or emphasising an aspect of concern to the group. A tradition may be strongly positioned within the discipline by the practice orientation or research findings of the founding genera- tion of leaders. Being values-based and genealogical, traditions can endure over many generations: this endurance often is expressed in political action in pursuit of values shared by the members.

A tradition is visible in:

- a boundedness of the group
- shared values, vocabulary, orientations to practice, research and teaching
- an explicit genealogy of personalised knowledge (teacher/student histories, collegial working, textual citation and oral references, research paradigms)
- honorific occasions, publications, ancestor-worship, folklore.

Influence

This seemed fairly obvious when we set out. We will, however, reflect further on 'influence' in Chapter 11 and in the Conclusion. According to this interpretative framework for *The Field of Knowledge*, we anticipated the field as a competitive influence field (like Darwin's Galapagos Islands, where different forms of life compete and some survive).

The influence–school/tradition–discipline–institution matrix is not a grid but a spiral, widening as it rises from influence → institution. Thus the higher up the spiral, the more control one has over bringing one's own professional knowledge into the field (though the more impersonal that knowledge has to be). The theoretical–practical/personal–political matrix provides the framework within which the dynamics of knowledge are made visible. What has to be thought of in relation to all these is knowledge.

With regard to influence, the mode of knowledge/form of influence is conversa- tion/al, rhetoric (as the intellectual tool and form). It is like a Jackson Pollock painting: lots of little splashes of individuals influencing others, whether patients or other nurses. There is mutuality: at this level everybody can bid to make his/her knowledge accepted. Here nurses are continually interacting with non- discipline-specific knowledge (of patients, of common sense). The mode is per- suasion, personal persuasion.

The membrane between influence and school/tradition is semi-permeable. Here one finds models, and the influence of some individuals becomes more discern- able. Knowledge is communicated by, e.g. the public lecture. However, it is not just a question of communicating knowledge when you are building a school, but also of sharing values, celebrating the group, being publicly thankful for leadership and acknowledging intellectual and professional indebtedness, con- firming that some are in and some are definitely out. To the cognitive is added the affective, but it is all more public than the process at the influence level. It is an exercise in building critical mass, giving people something to join. In Mary Douglas's terms (Douglas 1973: 77–92), it is group rather than grid (which is much more the habitat of the discipline). Still, rhetoric and persuasion are modes of knowledge transmission/forms of influence.

Regarding discipline, the communication is by books, texts. The mode/form of influence (perhaps, rather, the sign of disciplinary success from a sociology of knowledge point of view) is the paradigm. The paradigm is built by competition, and in principle there should be only one dominant paradigm in each area of knowledge. This can also include, e.g., the one-to-one relationship (as in Peplau's widely seen and influential film *Nurse–Patient Relationship*) or the group meeting – both forms of practice-embedded knowledge. This is also the point where the knowledge of users and 'sad people' comes in from outside the field – tubes, as it were, run from the field to outside it and vice versa.

Regarding institution, the mode is laws, codes, protocols, objectivity, truth, incontestable knowledge, the canon. The institution may be seen as seeking to impose a practice – based on 'science' – which competes with practice knowledge which is more *ad hoc*, occasioned, circumstantial, 'art'. The influence of institutions over individuals is complex, as it is more than knowledge that mediates this dominance: it is also legal orders, social control systems, custodial technology.

Tilley circulated this framework to the UK authors, saying that they could use it in considering how to write their chapters, but that they need not do so, and were free to write in the form they thought appropriate. In the Conclusion Tilley will consider both the extent to which we used it in our own contributions to the book, and also how other authors did or did not use it.

References

Altschul, A. (1997) A personal view of psychiatric nursing. In: *The Mental Health Nurse: Views of Practice and Education* (ed. S. Tilley), pp. 1–14. Oxford: Blackwell Science.

Barker, P. (1991) Finding common ground. *Nursing Times*, 87 (2): 37–8.

Barker, P.J. & Reynolds, B. (1996) Rediscovering the proper focus of nursing: a critique of Gournay's position on nursing theory and models. *Journal of Psychiatric and Mental Health Nursing*, 3 (1): 76–80.

Barker, P., Glenister, D., Jackson, S., *et al.* (2001) 'End of the old peer show?' *Mental Health Practice*, 1 (7): 22.

Berger, P.L. & Luckmann, T. (1971) *The Social Construction of Reality: A Treatise in the Sociology of Knowledge*. Harmondsworth: Penguin.

Blankenship, J. (1989) 'Magic' and 'mystery': in the works of Kenneth Burke. In: *The Legacy of Kenneth Burke* (eds H.W. Simons & T. Melia), pp. 128–51. Madison: University of Wisconsin Press.

Burns, T. (1969) On the plurality of social systems. In: *Industrial Man* (ed. T. Burns), pp. 232–49. Harmondsworth: Penguin.

Department of Health (1997) *The New NHS*. London: HMSO.

Douglas, M. (1973) *Natural Symbols: Explorations in Cosmology*. Harmondsworth: Penguin Books.

Doyle McCarthy, E. (1996) *Knowledge as Culture: The New Sociology of Knowledge*. London: Routledge.

Emerson, R.W. (1841) Circles. In: Emerson (1982) *Selected Essays* (edited and with an introduction by L. Ziff), pp. 225–38. Harmondsworth: Penguin.

Gournay, K. (1995) What to do with nursing models. *Journal of Psychiatric and Mental Health Nursing*, 2 (5): 325–7.

Gournay, K. (1997) Responses to 'What to do with nursing models' – a reply from Gournay. *Journal of Psychiatric and Mental Health Nursing*, 4 (3): 227–31.

Gournay, K. & Ritter, S. (1998) What future for research in mental health nursing: rejoinder to Parsons, Beech and Rolfe. *Journal of Psychiatric and Mental Health Nursing*, 5: 227–30.

Hodgkin, R.A. (1997) Making space for meaning. *Oxford Review of Education*, 23 (4): 385–99.

Lego, S. (1997) A critique of Gournay's position on nursing theory and models. *Journal of Psychiatric and Mental Health Nursing*, 4 (1): 64–6.

Parsons, S. (1997) The methodology of choice: a reply to Gournay and Ritter. *Journal of Psychiatric and Mental Health Nursing*, 4: 442–3.

Rolfe, G. (1996) What to do with psychiatric nursing. *Journal of Psychiatric and Mental Health Nursing*, 3 (5): 331–3.

Rolfe, G. (1997) Knowledge, power and authority: a response to Gournay and Ritter. *Journal of Psychiatric and Mental Health Nursing*, 4: 444–6.

Rolfe, G. (1998) The marriage of heaven and hell: further remarks on the future for mental health research. *Journal of Psychiatric and Mental Health Nursing*, 5: 230–33.

Szasz, T. (1979) *The Myth of Psychotherapy: Mental Healing as Religion, Rhetoric and Repression*. Oxford: Oxford University Press.

Tilley, S. (ed.) (1997) *The Mental Health Nurse: Views of Practice and Education*. Oxford: Blackwell Science.

Section 2

Looking Across the Field: Case Studies of Institutionalisation of Knowledge of Psychiatric and Mental Health Nursing

Chapter 2

The Institute of Psychiatry: Nursing within the Health Services Research Department

Kevin Gournay

Introduction

It would be very tempting to start this chapter by relating the history of nursing at the Royal Bethlem and Maudsley Hospital. Since the foundation of the Institute of Psychiatry in 1948, as a post-graduate medical school, clinical and academic activities of the Institute of Psychiatry and these hospitals have been inextricably linked, and this linkage continues to the present day. Indeed, since 1948 the Institute of Psychiatry has provided the academic base for psychiatrists and clinical psychologists working in those hospitals. Nursing, however, has had a different history from these other care professions for a variety of reasons. The nurse training school at the Bethlem and Maudsley hospitals was of course enormously influential in a number of ways, not least in the number of very important international figures who are associated with it. Since World War II these figures have included Eileen Skellern, the Chief Nursing Officer, and Professor Annie Altschul, who conducted what were arguably the first high quality psychiatric nursing research studies in the UK. Nursing education remained within the Maudsley hospital until 1987, when the Institute of Psychiatry inaugurated a Section of Psychiatric Nursing, and appointed the first Senior Lecturer in psychiatric nursing, Dr Julia Brooking. Julia not only occupied the position of academic nursing lead within the Institute, but also was Chief Nursing Officer for the Royal Bethlem and Maudsley Hospitals. In the years after Julia's arrival at the Institute, the move of nursing into higher education began, and by the mid 1990s pre-registration education moved from the Maudsley Hospital to the Nursing Department at King's College (now the Nightingale Institute) and to the South Bank Polytechnic, now the South Bank University. Post-registration courses (some of which will be referred to in detail below) eventually became educational programmes of the Institute of Psychiatry, and by the time I arrived at the Institute in 1995, the Bethlem and Maudsley Hospitals had no formal pre-registration training for psychiatric nurses of its own. Since 1995 the Bethlem and Maudsley Hospitals have been incorporated into the South London and Maudsley NHS Trust, an enormous organisation with an operating budget of £200 million and a workforce of four thousand, of whom two and a half thousand are psychiatric nurses. The Trust catchment area now spreads across four boroughs of south-east London, and includes more than one hundred sites for clinical services, including not only the Bethlem and Maudsley Hospitals but also the psychiatric departments in St Thomas's Hospital, Guy's Hospital, King's College Hospital, the Mayday Hospital in Croydon and a wide array of specialist and generic teams situated throughout the community.

As noted above, it would be tempting to provide much more by way of histor-ical backdrop, but for the purposes of this book it is probably most important to describe the contemporary scene. The Chair of Psychiatric Nursing at the Insti-tute of Psychiatry was inaugurated in 1995, largely as a result of the efforts of Professor Sir David Goldberg, who was Professor of Psychiatry at the Institute from 1993 until 1999. By Sir David's account (and, indeed, this is a view shared by many others), in 1993 the Institute was the world's leading research institu-tion in mental health, but was also regarded as an iconoclastic institution, which had only three significant disciplines, i.e. psychiatry, clinical psychology and basic neuroscience. While it is true that at the time of Sir David's arrival, nursing, social work and the other disciplines were represented by various junior mem-bers of Institute staff, there was very little significant research or teaching activity by these 'peripheral' disciplines. Indeed, the outside mental health community heavily criticised the Institute for its lack of relevance to the modern National Health Service. As Director of Research and Development for the then Bethlem and Maudsley Trust, Sir David began a number of initiatives aimed at producing a truly multidisciplinary approach to the problems of modern mental health care. He also set about developing the conditions of infrastructure that would enable the Institute to build research programmes that have real relevance to the NHS, and to the lives of real people. As part of the strategy Sir David put in place the measures necessary to recruit leaders in other disciplines and by his efforts my Chair in Psychiatric Nursing was inaugurated in 1995. At the same time, a Chair in Mental Health Economics was inaugurated and filled by Professor Martin Knapp. More recently a Chair of Social Work was inaugurated and filled by Professor Peter Huxley, Sir David's long-time collaborator in Manchester and, without doubt, one of the most well-known psychiatric social workers in the world. Shortly after my arrival Sir David set in place other initiatives which were to result in the founding of a brand new department, the Health Services Research Department, whereby all of the health services research expertise of the Institute was concentrated in one location rather than being spread out across a number of disparate research groups.

By 1999, Sir David's efforts had resulted in the funding for a new building for health services research, very appropriately named the David Goldberg Centre; this opened its doors in February 2001. This was far from being a tokenistic effort to demonstrate that the Institute was at least multidisciplinary in name; Sir David also ensured that Martin Knapp, Peter Huxley and I were placed in positions where we could exert real influence for change. In my own case, I was appointed Chair of the Institute's Academic Board in 1997 for a two-year period. This com-mittee was, at that time, the centrepiece of the Institute's management. As Chair of the Academic Board I was privy to every top-level strategic initiative as well as consulted about each and every important activity within all of the Institute departments, and indeed within the Trust. Sir David ensured that others (including myself) were placed in real positions of influence on initiatives that included the reshaping of education and the foundation of various interdisciplinary research groups across the Institute. Sir David also encouraged all Health Services Research staff to develop and improve the Institute's relationship with the Government via its links with the Department of Health. Thus, I have no reservations in commencing this chapter by saying that the recent growth of psychiatric nursing within the Institute has been largely the responsibility of Sir David Goldberg. His vision has included each and every discipline playing its part in the development of an organisation that would, through research, yield new knowledge, and through its education strategies disseminate that new knowledge and the accompanying skills to the workforce. I believe that it is important to emphasise that the philosophy of those within the Institute who have a psychiatric nursing background is that psychiatric nursing knowledge should be seen as but one component of a wider body of knowledge shared by other disciplines. It is at the same time an area that can only develop within partnerships which include other professions, consumers, carers and, indeed, the general public.

It is also worth noting that since my appointment at the Institute, there has been a reasonably close working relationship with colleagues in the Nightingale Institute at King's College, London. Collaboration with colleagues within nursing at King's has been strengthened by the integration of the Institute of Psychiatry as a school within King's College. However, the nurses within the Institute took the decision to keep the activities of psychiatric nursing within the Institute separate from those of our general nursing colleagues at King's (and indeed the mental health nurses in that department). This decision was based on the overall strategy of keeping psychiatric nursing within a broad multidisciplinary group, rather than have it join a 'nursing family'. A sign of the extent of cohesion of our research grouping at the Institute is that we have only one entry into the Research Assessment Exercise, covering all disciplines, and in the latest Exercise in 2001 we were rated 5* [note: the highest possible rating]. As noted above, we believe that nursing activities should be part of an overall integrated approach rather than attempting to develop research and education and training as a primarily unidisciplinary activity.

Current contributions to psychiatric nursing knowledge

How, therefore, is the group of psychiatric nurses at the Institute contributing to psychiatric nursing knowledge? Taken as given the view that psychiatric nursing knowledge should be located within a broad range of knowledge shared by other members of the mental health community, our overall philosophy has been underpinned by the recognition that as a discipline, psychiatric nursing is in need of considerable development. For at least five years the main aims of the Psychiatric

Nursing group within the Institute have been explicit, and focus on six areas, which have a considerable degree of overlap. The aims of this group are:

(1) To carry out high quality research which has a focus on important nursing topics which may also have multidisciplinary relevance
(2) To carry out research that is relevant to the development of mental health policy
(3) To provide assistance to Government in developing various policy initiatives across health care
(4) To develop a critical mass of a suitably-trained research workforce of individuals from a psychiatric nursing background
(5) To develop, test and disseminate innovative programmes of education and training to the nursing and more general health workforce
(6) To provide input to various service developments within both local and national services, and to disseminate research findings into everyday clinical practice.

Prior to providing some detail of how we are setting out to deliver these aims, and at the risk of some repetition, it is worth emphasising that in order to achieve these aims we have needed the support and collaboration of a wide range of individuals from different professions. Thus, for example, all of our major research projects have very close collaboration with world-class statisticians, health economists and epidemiologists. Similarly, whilst many projects are led by psychiatric nurses who hold and manage the grants, there is always, in these projects, substantial involvement from colleagues from other backgrounds and disciplines who bring particular expertise to relevant areas.

Following a description of our progress in delivering the above aims, I discuss how we intend to use a recently published framework for complex health interventions, which is being used by the Medical Research Council as a template for future research and dissemination.

High quality research

Our overall priority has been to focus our research efforts on evaluations of service and training programmes using the highest quality research methodologies. At the heart of our strategy has been the use of the randomised controlled trial. However, in juxtaposition to the randomised controlled trial we have used other research methods within the same project. For example, we have included economic analyses and various qualitative strategies. Furthermore, as we shall show below, we have on occasion used epidemiological methods to support our research. Whilst there has been a great deal of discussion in the nursing literature which has questioned the use of the randomised controlled trial, it seems to us that these arguments are vacuous. All of the major funding agencies, Government itself and scientific communities worldwide are in agreement that the randomised controlled trial is the gold standard for assessing effectiveness. Nevertheless, it is worth noting that although there is general agreement in accepting the randomised controlled trial as the gold standard, there are two important additional issues to note.

The first is that there are, of course, randomised controlled trials of excellent quality and those of poor quality, and there is little doubt that in the past undue weighting has been placed on the results of poorly designed trials carried out in mental health.

The second issue concerns qualitative research. It seems clear that overall, qualitative methods have in the past been greatly undervalued, and within psychiatric nursing there is obviously a place for such studies. However, we would also argue that there have been several difficulties regarding the use of qualitative methods within psychiatric nursing research.

The first point to make is that many qualitative researchers (like many quantitative researchers) have taken a completely polarised view of the area, and been unable to accept that other methods are of value.

The second point to make is that qualitative studies carried out in isolation yield only very limited knowledge. Furthermore, it is clear that qualitative strategies are greatly enhanced by placing them in juxtaposition to quantitative outcomes and/or developing the qualitative findings into more generalisable concepts. To take two simple examples, simply obtaining the views of mental health consumers during the process of care is not enough. It is important to understand how perceptions relate to the outcomes of the process of care, in terms of improvements or otherwise in symptoms and social functioning. To take this one stage further, we know from many studies (e.g. Gournay and Brooking 1994) that satisfaction with treatment as rated by the patient does not necessarily correlate with improvement on outcome measures of symptom or disability. With regard to using qualitative findings to generate something more generalisable, the example of the Camberwell Assessment of Need (Phelan *et al.* 1995) is most illustrative. This instrument, which has now been translated into dozens of languages, measures met and unmet needs, as defined by the user, the carer and the professional concerned. This instrument covers a range of areas including occupation, housing and social life.

Third, our somewhat negative view of qualitative research has been reinforced by the fact that much research carried out by psychiatric nurses is arguably of extremely poor quality, and one must cite the damning evidence of the last Research Assessment Exercise as confirming this.

Finally one also needs to make the point that many of the qualitative researchers who object to randomised controlled trials are individuals who have never received more than a derisory amount of training in quantitative methods. It is sadly true that psychiatric nursing academics at the most senior level have often been elevated to professorial positions within months or at most a few years after obtaining a PhD carried out in a very narrow area. It would be very interesting to examine the amount of research training obtained by senior academics in psychiatric nursing, and compare this research training with that of colleagues from other professions. Simply put, one may draw the conclusion that the criticism of quantitative research, and randomised controlled trials in particular, may be born of ignorance and a total lack of experience of these methods rather than any robust set of arguments.

Since 1995 the volume of research grants that support the nursing-focused projects at the Institute has now reached more than £3 million, and the largest of our studies have concentrated on workforce skills. For example, during 2000 we completed a randomised controlled trial to assess the training provided to practice nurses to detect and manage mental health problems in primary care. This study involved 36 general practices and over 4000 patients spread over a variety of rural, suburban and urban areas (preliminary results have been reported in Plummer *et al.* 2000). In an area related to core psychiatric nursing skills we also have been involved in examining medication management from a number of perspectives. As part of the background work, we have conducted Cochrane reviews on depot medication for schizophrenia, and carried out a specific Cochrane review regarding patient and nurse perspectives (Walburn *et al.* 2001) and collaborated in broader reviews of effectiveness (Quraishi and David 2000). Recently we completed a randomised controlled trial that evaluated a package of training in medication management for community psychiatric nurses working in various clinical services in different parts of the country (Gray 2001). This study showed that 80 hours of training in medication management leads to significant changes in the skills and knowledge of community psychiatric nurses (CPNs), but perhaps more importantly leads to clinically significant improvements in the conditions of the patients that they care for. This exploratory trial served as the basis of the funding we received from the Medical Research Council (MRC) to conduct a definitive trial of medication management (Gray *et al.* 2003). Our approach to medication management research is therefore very much in line with the recently published MRC framework for the evaluation of complex health interventions (Campbell *et al.* 2000) to which we will refer below. At the time of writing we have now extended this research on medication management to a five-country study funded by the European Union (1.7 million Euros). The data collection for this study will be complete by November 2004, with results being published over the next year.

Our other research programmes include work on people with challenging behaviour and learning disabilities, the use of cognitive behavioural interventions in primary care and studies to which we will refer below which have been funded as part of research training fellowships. The other main study worth describing is soon to be completed. This is a randomised controlled trial of training in dual diagnosis interventions. This work developed as a result of our interest in training staff in an integrated approach towards the problems of serious mental illness and substance abuse. We developed our first modules of training in 1997. Following the piloting of this training, a consideration of the literature (Gournay *et al.* 1997) and some baseline epidemiological work (Menezes *et al.* 1996; Wright *et al.* 2000), we obtained funding for a randomised controlled trial of training. This study involves 74 case managers. Our primary outcomes are the clinical, social functioning and economic outcomes of some 200 patients with dual diagnosis who were case managed by these workers (about half of the case managers are nurses). This study extends across a large area of south-east London and includes case managers working in no less than 11 community health centres. As well as patient outcomes, we have also measured the impact of training on the case managers in terms of skill and knowledge.

Research relevant to mental health policy

Over the past five years, our policy research efforts have been wide-ranging and we have carried out several surveys relevant to mental health policy to support various national policy initiatives. These include: a national survey of practice nurses, particularly examining the quantity and nature of their mental health interventions and their training needs (Gray *et al.* 1999); a national follow-up of all nurse therapists trained on the ENB 650 (Cognitive Behavioural Therapy) course 1972 (Gournay *et al.* 2000); two surveys of the training of staff in the management of violence (Gournay 2001; Lee *et al.* 2001); and the survey of Trust policies in the management of violence (Noak *et al.* 2002). In addition we have carried out a one-day census of wards in 12 inner London mental health services, specifically focusing on nursing issues (Gournay *et al.* 1997). This work on inpatient wards was used to underpin the report on inpatient care *Addressing Acute Concerns*, published by the Department of Health in 1999 (DoH 1999). We have also completed research for the Workforce Action Team of the National Service Framework for Mental Health, which sets out to map the capacity of the English university system to deliver training necessary to meet National Service Framework priorities (Brooker *et al.* 2000). The above are some examples of the studies we have completed. In addition we have conducted other work on suicide, primary care and NHS Direct.

We believe that this policy-related research, while somewhat limited in its scientific quality, is important as it provides some cross-sectional views of the state of mental health services. With the setting up of the recently announced National Institute for Mental Health (England), such policy-related research is of vital importance. This Institute will be formed in part by a network of the leading mental health institutions and the role of Departments such as ours in developing policy will become a much greater priority. Given that mental health nurses are the largest workforce in mental health care, surveys that provide a picture of skills, practice and training are very relevant to developing nursing-related policies.

Providing assistance to Government in developing policy initiatives

Simply put, this area covers our efforts to disseminate the results of research (our own and others) to Government departments and to assist Government in understanding how this research should inform policy. As noted above, we were commissioned to carry out various surveys, which have subsequently influenced policy, but we have also taken part in the actual process of developing the Government policies by taking on work within committees, task forces and working groups.

Various members of the department have provided literature reviews, scoping studies and thematic reviews for civil servants and ministers. Recently we conducted thematic reviews of research priorities linked to the National Plan and National Service Framework, research priorities in inpatient mental health care, a review of stress in forensic mental health nurses and reviews relating to primary care. We have also contributed to a number of committees including the two Clinical Standards Advisory Group Committees on depression and schizophrenia. We have had substantial input into the reference group for the National Service Framework, the clinical systems initiative, the Workforce Action Team of the National Service Framework and the nursing strategy for England, as well as a wide range of committees set up by Government and other organisations such as the Sainsbury Centre for Mental Health.

One other way that policy initiatives may be assisted is by the development of debate and discussion. In 1997, Sir David Goldberg set about producing a publication stream which he hoped would influence debate in mental health care regarding important and controversial topics. To this end, the Maudsley Discussion Paper series was launched. By mid-2001, 11 discussion papers had been published on a range of important topics including child and adolescent mental health services, special hospitals and the implementation of community approaches for people with serious mental illness. The first and eleventh discussion papers have had a major focus on mental health nursing. The first discussion paper, *The GP, the Psychiatrist and the Burden of Mental Health Care* (Goldberg and Gournay 1997), reviewed the problems associated with mental health in primary care and set out an agenda for improving access to a high quality mental health service, for the very large number of people with mental health problems. This paper has been used as a discussion document within the Department of Health and has recently proved to be very influential in the development of the National Service Framework for Mental Health. More recently, a discussion paper entitled *Should Mental Health Nurses Prescribe?* (Gournay and Gray 2001) responded to the Government consultation exercise on nurse prescribing and reviewed the options for mental health nurses. The discussion paper concluded that providing mental health nurses with prescriptive authority was likely to be a positive development, but added that caution was essential. In particular, the discussion paper, in its review of evidence, highlighted the importance of comprehensive programmes of education and training and rigorous evaluation of these programmes within the context of multi-centre randomised controlled trials. Such research will hopefully show that providing mental health nurses with prescriptive authority will be generalisable across different parts of the country. This discussion paper series is set to continue and there is no doubt that mental health nursing will be a topic on which the series will focus time and time again, and this will provide another method for the development of knowledge.

The development of a critical mass of individuals from a psychiatric nursing background suitably trained in research

The Government has recognised that there are substantial challenges to be faced in providing a sufficient infrastructure to carry out nursing research. These are set out in a discussion paper (DoH 2000). As noted above, it is our view that it is essential that we build capacity by providing research training to individuals from a psychiatric nursing background at both pre- and post-doctoral level. As a corollary of our efforts we have recently set up a multidisciplinary training programme (at Masters level) in mental health services research, which will be the first of its kind anywhere in the world. This course has modules covering the entire range of research methods and we are very fortunate to have our programme linked with those of the London School for Hygiene and Tropical Medicine and the Johns Hopkins Institute in Baltimore. We believe that our trainee researchers need to be nourished in a multidisciplinary environment which covers a range of disciplines including statistics, health economics, epidemiology and social science. We also take the view that trainee researchers need to be close to a variety of research programmes which include the widest range of methods possible. Siting research training in large multidisciplinary departments allows our trainee researchers continuous exposure to colleagues carrying out a wide range of research (approximately 120 projects currently funded through our department). We have funding for seven Research Training Fellowships for people from a nursing background including three post-doctoral Fellowships. Funding bodies include the Department of Health, the Welsh Assembly and the Medical Research Council.

It is our view that the task of developing a suitably-sized mental health nursing research workforce will take more than a decade. Ideally, we need to recruit from people who are young enough to have the requisite energy and enthusiasm, but who also are experienced enough to clearly understand the context in which they are developing their skills. One of the obstacles that will face us and which we have already encountered in our work at the Institute is that of financial reward. Our trainee researchers will be paid on the scales equivalent to that of University Lecturer and be required to demonstrate considerable achievements in terms of publication in high quality peer review journals and the acquisition of research grants of their own, before they can be promoted to Senior Lecturer. The salary scales for Lecturer and Senior Lecturer compare badly with the salary scale for Nurse Consultant and we are increasingly finding that our research trainees could, if they so wished, obtain nurse consultant posts without any difficulty. This situation is similar to that found in medicine where trainee researchers with a medical background are often gravely disadvantaged. Thus we have junior researchers who are qualified psychiatrists, being paid on salary scales that are between £10 000 and £15 000 less than they would obtain in the NHS. More senior doctors undertaking post-doctoral research training are even more disadvantaged. The Department of Health has recognised the problems of properly-rewarded career pathways and it seems likely that the Government will introduce improvements which will keep people within research careers. Unless this is done, nursing as well as the other disciplines will suffer, we will not be able to achieve the critical mass needed and this will have obvious implications for the future development of knowledge.

The development, testing and dissemination of innovative programmes of education and training

When I came to the Institute in 1995, I was fortunate to find that the basis for evidence-based education and training was long established. Indeed, I had myself trained on one of these evidence-based programmes in the 1970s (Joint Board of Clinical Nursing Studies Course 650 – Adult Behavioural Psychotherapy; first established in 1972). In addition, the Thorn Programme, training nurses in evidence-based interventions for serious mental illness, has been running since 1992 and I was fortunate to have been the external examiner for this course between 1992 and 1995. Using these two programmes as a base, we have subsequently developed other evidence-based training in dual diagnosis, medication management, family interventions in schizophrenia, acute inpatient care, practice nursing, community forensic care and other related programmes. We have all put enormous efforts into the dissemination of our training programmes throughout the NHS and wider. Fortunately, we were provided with resources to expand these efforts by a very large personal financial contribution from Dr Jim Birley, former Dean of the Institute and one of the main figures behind the development of the Thorn Programme at the Institute and the University of Manchester. In all, our training has reached no fewer than 55 Trusts across the NHS and we have been instrumental in setting up no fewer than 12 programmes in other universities in the UK. Our training efforts have also extended to other parts of Europe and Australia and we are now in the midst of developing programmes for various parts of the former Soviet Union and South America.

Our emphasis has been on disseminating training based on hard evidence and thus our focus has been on Cognitive Behavioural Therapy, Assertive Community Treatment and other psychosocial interventions. As noted above, we have also tested training by randomised controlled trial and we believe that our educational efforts in medication management, dual diagnosis and mental health interventions for practice nurses probably represent the first attempts to research educational programmes using the randomised controlled trial on large numbers of nurses. We have made the point over and over again (e.g. Gournay and Thornicroft 2000) that while literally millions of pounds are expended on training throughout the NHS, few if any resources are deployed to evaluate the outcome of such training. We are pleased to note that the new National Institute for Mental Health will, as part of its core function, ensure that the evaluation of training is central in the research agenda.

The new National Institute of Mental Health has as one of its core functions the development of suitable training programmes for the NHS. It is therefore of vital importance that mental health nursing begins to adopt a much more unified approach to training. The partnerships that will be forged within the National Institute for Mental Health will surely be positive, as we will be able to share expertise. Between various university providers, we are likely to see a concentration of efforts on evidence-based courses and hopefully this emphasis will generalise rapidly to pre-registration programmes.

Providing input to service developments within local and national services

As was noted at the beginning of this chapter, the Institute of Psychiatry's activities are inextricably linked with those of the South London and Maudsley NHS Trust. This has obviously helped ensure that the nurses of the Health Services Research Department have a robust clinical as well as academic focus. This is clearly advantageous in a world where academic nursing is often largely divorced from mainstream NHS activity and where applying the results of academic endeavours into clinical practice are often compromised by the distance between university and NHS providers. Obviously, much of the research activity detailed above is carried out within the Trust. However, in addition, we have facilitated a number of practice developments outwith the Trust. Notable among these are the development of a depression walk-in clinic, funded by the Charlie Waller Memorial Trust at the London Region Office of the NHS, and the application of computer-based treatment programmes in Cognitive Behavioural Therapy. Also as noted above, our training programmes have reached more than 55 Trusts across England; we have also carried out on-site training in Scotland, Wales and Northern Ireland, as well as setting up programmes in Irish and Welsh Universities. More widely, we have been involved in a range of initiatives run by the World Health Organization (WHO). Fortunately for us, the Institute of Psychiatry is a WHO-collaborating centre, and under the leadership of Professor Rachel Jenkins there is a substantial network of WHO activities within the Department, including not only training initiatives, but also policy development and human rights activities.

It is also worth noting that each year we receive in the Institute literally hundreds of international visitors. We are pleased that there are now growing numbers of nurses from Africa, the USA, Europe, Australasia and other parts of the world who visit our Department for periods from a few hours to several months. We are delighted that we have now established some of our visitors with honorary Institute appointments. The most notable of these is a visiting professorship for Gail Stuart, arguably one of the most important psychiatric nurses of the last two decades, who holds an appointment at the Medical University of South Carolina.

Framework for the future development of nursing activities within the Health Services Research Department

Recently, the MRC published a framework which offers a structure to the chain of events from initial idea to dissemination of proven intervention and can be seen as a parallel to the five phases recognised in the development of pharmaceutical interventions (see Fig. 2.1).

As the figure shows, there are five phases, which set out the process for the development-testing and dissemination of knowledge. We believe that this framework has enormous implications for mental health nursing. We would argue that, so far, much nursing research has focused on only fragments of this framework. There have, for example, been endless explorations of relevant theory, but there has been little attempt to operationalise the active components of interventions. This identification process is the second phase of the MRC model. As the subsequent phases of the model show, there is a need then to follow a logical process which involves testing within the confines of an experimental procedure, then the replication of the intervention within ordinary settings, and finally replicating the intervention over all services. The state of knowledge in mental health care compared with other medical disciplines is poor and Lewis and colleagues in an editorial in *Psychological Medicine* describe the task of having definitive evidence to cover mental health care as Herculean (Lewis *et al.* 1997). At the present time, the only interventions in mental health care with a well-developed background theory are psychological interventions such as Cognitive Behavioural Therapy. We obviously need to continue with our attempts to develop a theoretical understanding of what components of mental health nursing are effective. Simply put, it is our view that we should start almost with a *tabula rasa* and cast aside various archaic theories which continue to preoccupy many nursing academics and which are merely a source of frustration. With regard to the exploratory trials referred to in the framework, the work of Charlie Brooker and colleagues (Brooker *et al.* 1994) was an excellent example of what can be achieved within limited resources. Charlie's work, as I wish to record here, has been one of the influences in encouraging us to develop exploratory trials. With regard to definitive trials, as noted above, we are now beginning to work on these within specified areas and not until much more work of this variety has been undertaken will we be able to do justice to the area of dissemination. However, we feel that we are beginning to disseminate some evidence-based methods to the NHS, but, as noted above, in several other areas our aims and aspirations need to be cast over a long period; certainly a decade and probably much longer.

Conclusion

The group of nurses who work within the Health Services Research Department at the Institute of Psychiatry probably constitute the largest grouping of psychiatric nurses engaged in research in any country outside of the USA. In several

Theory	Modelling	Exploratory trial	Definitive randomised controlled trial	Long-term implementation
Explore relevant theory to ensure best choice of intervention and hypothesis and to predict major confounders and strategic design issues	Identify the components of the intervention, and the underlying mechanisms by which they will influence outcomes to provide evidence that you can predict how they relate to and interact with each other	Describe the constant and variable components of a replicable intervention *and* a feasible protocol for comparing the intervention with an appropriate alternative	Compare a fully defined intervention with an appropriate alternative using a protocol that is theoretically defensible, reproducible and adequately controlled, in a study with appropriate statistical power	Determine whether others can reliably replicate your intervention and results in uncontrolled settings over the long term
Pre-clinical	**Phase I**	**Phase II**	**Phase III**	**Phase IV**

Fig. 2.1 Interventions to improve health. (From Campbell *et al.* 2000).

places these nurses work within a truly multidisciplinary team and do not form in any sense a department or entity of their own. Nevertheless, we believe that this grouping of nurses does provide knowledge that is essential to the nursing function within mental health services. At the level of providing new scientific knowledge, we believe that we have demonstrated a formidable track record, exemplified in our numerous publications in high quality peer-reviewed journals, as well as our embryonic efforts within the Cochrane collaboration. Perhaps the largest challenge as with any groups of researchers within mental health care is to actually influence clinical practice. While our efforts in this regard are substantial, it would be premature indeed to suggest that these efforts have yielded real changes in clinical areas at local, national and international levels. Only time will tell how successful we have been.

References

Brooker, C., Falloon, I., Butterworth, A., Goldberg, D., Graham-Hole, V. & Hillier, V. (1994) The outcome of training community psychiatric nurses to deliver psychosocial intervention. *British Journal of Psychiatry*, 160: 836–44.

Brooker, C., Gournay, K., O'Halloran, P. & Bailey, D. (2000) *Mapping the Capacity of the English University System to Deliver NSF Priorities*. Report to the Workforce Action Team. London: DoH.

Campbell, M., Fitzpatrick, R., Haines, A., *et al.* (2000) Framework for design and evaluation of complex interventions to improve health. *British Medical Journal*, 321: 694–97.

DoH (1999) *Addressing Acute Concerns*. Report of the Standing Nursing Midwifery Advisory Committee. London: DoH.

DoH (2000) *Consultation Paper on the Future of Nursing Research*. London: DoH.

Goldberg, D. & Gournay, K. (1997) *The GP, the Psychiatrist and the Burden of Mental Health Care*, Maudsley Discussion Paper No. 1. London: Institute of Psychiatry.

Gournay, K. (2001) *The Prevention, Recognition and Management of Violence in Mental Health Care*. Report to the UKCC. London: UKCC.

Gournay, K. & Brooking, J. (1994) Community psychiatric nurses in primary health care. *British Journal of Psychiatry*, 165: 231–8.

Gournay, K. & Gray, R. (2001) *Should Mental Health Nurses Prescribe?* Maudsley Discussion Paper No. 11. London: Institute of Psychiatry.

Gournay, K. & Thornicroft, G. (2000) Comments on the UK700 case management trial. *British Journal of Psychiatry*, 177: 371.

Gournay, K., Sandford, T., Thornicroft, G. & Johnson, S. (1997) Training and service delivery in dual diagnosis: a challenge for nursing. *Journal of Psychiatric and Mental Health Nursing*, 4: 89–95.

Gournay, K., Denford, L., Parr, A. & Newell, R. (2000) British nurses in behavioural psychotherapy: a 25 year follow-up. *Journal of Advanced Nursing*, 32 (2): 343–51.

Gray, R. (2001) *A Randomised Controlled Trial of Training CPN's in Medication Management*. PhD Thesis, University of London.

Gray, R., Parr, A., Plummer, S., *et al.* (1999) A national survey of practice nurse involvement with mental health interventions. *Journal of Advanced Nursing*, 30 (4): 901–906.

Gray, R., Wykes, T. & Gournay, K. (2003) Effectiveness of medication management training on community mental health nursing skills. *International Journal of Nursing Studies*, 40 (2): 163–169.

Lee, S., Wright, S., Sayer, J., Parr, A., Gray, R. & Gournay, K. (2001) Physical restraint training for nurses in English and Welsh psychiatric intensive care and regional secure units. *Journal of Mental Health*, 10 (2): 151–162.

Lewis, G., Churchill, R. & Hotopf, M. (1997) Editorial: systematic reviews and meta-analysis. *Psychological Medicine*, 27: 3–7.

Menezes, P., Johnson, S. & Thornicroft, G. (1996) Drug and alcohol problems among individuals with severe mental illness in south London. *British Journal of Psychiatry*, 169: 334–7.

Noak, J., Wright, S., Sayer, J., *et al.* (2002) The content of management of violence policy documents in United Kingdom Mental Health Units. *Journal of Advanced Nursing*, 37: 294–301.

Phelan, M., Slade, M. & Thornicroft, G. (1995) The Camberwell assessment of need. *British Journal of Psychiatry*, 167: 589–95.

Plummer, S., Mann, A., Ritter, S. & Gournay, K. (2000) Detection of psychological distress by practice nurses in general practice. *Psychological Medicine*, 30: 1233–7.

Quraishi, S. & David, A. (2000) *Depot Flupenthixol Decanoate for Schizophrenia or Other Psychotic Disorders*. Cochrane Library, Issue 2. Oxford: Update Software.

Walburn, J., Gray, R., Gournay, K., Quraifhi, S. & David, A. (2001) Systematic review of patient and nurse attitudes to depot medication. *British Journal of Psychiatry*, 179: 300–307.

Wright, S., Gournay, K., Glorney, E. & Thornicroft, G. (2000) Dual diagnosis in the suburbs: prevalence, need and inpatient service use. *Social Psychiatry and Psychiatric Epidemiology*, 35: 297–304.

Chapter 3

Fragile Tradition: Institutionalisation of Knowledge of Psychiatric and Mental Health Nursing in the Department of Nursing Studies, the University of Edinburgh

Stephen Tilley

> The history of a practice in our time is generally and characteristically embedded in and made intelligible in terms of the larger and longer history of the tradition through which the practice in its present form was conveyed to us. . . . (MacIntyre 1985: 222)

Introduction

In this chapter I offer an account of knowledge about psychiatric and mental health nursing[1], as institutionalised in practices of teaching, supervision and research in the Department of Nursing Studies, at the University of Edinburgh[2]. I will set the *present* practices in the context of the *tradition* of psychiatric and mental health nursing in the Department, using Alasdair MacIntyre's notions of 'practice' and 'tradition'.

By 'practice' MacIntyre means:

> . . . any coherent and complex form of socially established cooperative human activity through which goods internal to that form of activity are realized in the course of trying to achieve those standards of excellence which are appropriate to, and partially definitive of, that form of activity, with the result that human powers to achieve excellence, and

---

[1] The question of what to call the nurses whose title has changed over time, and who use different titles to signify important distinctions in the field, is problematic. I have chosen to use the term 'psychiatric and mental health nurse', as I think that the people so called may work under the auspices of psychiatry or psychiatric knowledge, but may also work under the auspices of mental health care and knowledge related thereto. This use is consistent with that in e.g., the *Journal of Psychiatric and Mental Health Nursing*.

[2] I will refer to what is now the School as 'the Department', for that was its name for most of its existence until recent reorganisation. Its designation prior to becoming a Department will be noted where relevant.

human conceptions of the ends and goods involved, are systematically extended. (MacIntyre 1985: 187)

He characterises 'tradition' as follows:

> A living tradition ... is an historically extended, socially embodied argument, and an argument precisely in part about the goods which constitute that tradition. (MacIntyre 1985: 222)

The claim of this chapter is that the scholarly *'practice'* central to the tradition is critical scholarly description and evaluation of psychiatric nursing practice. The scholarly practice as 'human activity' is 'socially embodied' or 'socially established' in teaching, supervision and research. The 'goods internal to' that *scholarly* practice are: (1) challenging psychiatric and mental health nurses to account for and argue about nursing practice in professional, policy and institutional contexts; (2) challenging them to change their practices in light of (1); and (3) challenging the basis of relationships in practice.[3] The 'human powers' and 'human conceptions of the ends and goods involved' are necessarily both those of this scholarly practice and those of the practice of psychiatric and mental health nursing. Internal to the scholarly practice is the good that its accounts extend the 'human powers' and 'human conceptions of the ends and goods involved' of both scholars *and* mental health nurses. For practitioners these powers and conceptions include e.g., powers of care, healing and therapy, to realise the end and good of development of *persons in relationship in community*; for scholars they include, e.g., powers of critical thinking and understanding.

The remainder of this chapter consists of four parts. First, an emblematic story illustrating the tradition's practices, ends and goods is presented, token of the larger 'story' of which those in the tradition are parts. Second, the 'original' institutional context of mental health nursing research and teaching in the University of Edinburgh is portrayed, to highlight the values-base of the tradition. Third, the three goods of scholarly practice noted above are discussed with reference to teaching, supervision and research. The fragility of the tradition is a constant theme, and the conclusions focus on the prospects for this fragile tradition as it confronts the discontinuities of volatile academic, institutional, professional and policy environments.

---

[3] The claim that the scholarly practice is socially embodied needs justification. Susan Sladden, one of those I count in the tradition, thinks that those I consider part of it may not necessarily all recognise themselves as such; that I have still to establish a coherent tradition existing outside my own imagination (Susan Sladden, personal communication). Furthermore, it is true that at any given time there have been few psychiatric and mental health nurse lecturers or researchers in the Department – sometimes one, often as at present two: a fragile line of descent. Nonetheless, I discern 'socially embodied cooperative activity' in the succession of higher degree supervision relationships, and in teaching and learning consciously based on reflexive social interaction and argument. My aim in this chapter is to substantiate this claim.

An emblematic story

The caption Annie Altschul, late Professor Emeritus in our Department, composed in 1999 to accompany her 80th-birthday portrait photograph[4] provides a key to understanding the tradition:

> Professor Emeritus Annie T. Altschul
> CBE BA MSc RGN RMN RNT FRCN
> Arriving in the UK in 1938 as a refugee from Nazi Austria, taking up Nursing was a natural option, **faute de mieux**. However, as soon as I discovered psychiatric nursing, I was sold on a career as a nurse. My passionate concern for people who suffer from mental disorder, my affinity with them and my quest for knowledge about mental illness has never flagged. In order to underpin my practice as a psychiatric nurse with better theoretical knowledge, while working at the Maudsley I embarked on simultaneous full-time study of Psychology at Birkbeck College, University of London.
>
> In 1964, it was my good fortune to join the staff in the fairly-recently established Department of Nursing Studies at The University of Edinburgh. Over a period of almost 20 years, until my retirement in 1983, I enjoyed the enormous benefits of the intellectual and academic stimulus provided by colleagues and students along with opportunities to research and to travel, and to contribute nationally and internationally to professional, political and scientific progress. After I had been promoted to the Chair of Nursing Studies in 1976, I discovered – with the help of colleagues and students – that there were many other interesting areas of nursing as well as my own!
>
> Psychiatric nursing does not lend itself to pictorial representation and so I chose to have this picture taken in my own home where I am surrounded by music and books, and where visitors are always welcome. The painting behind me forms a link with my origins: an Austrian rural dwelling with lilac, horse chestnut and window boxes – a painting which was the sole possession my mother decided to bring with her when she joined me in exile, now over 60 years ago.

Annie frames the story of herself in the Department of Nursing Studies within two other stories: the story of exile and the story of becoming a psychiatric nurse. Each story forms a context for understanding the others. Passionate concern for and affinity with those who suffer conjoin the stories of exile and psychiatric nursing. The quest for knowledge about mental illness is a line of continuity between the practitioner intent on extending theoretical knowledge and the scholar in the University. Together, the stories establish a hermeneutic of ethics and knowledge. They convey Annie's standpoint[5] as person-in-relationship, participating in and conjoining institutions and communities (of origin, of practice, academic,

---

[4] The photo with its caption hangs on the wall opposite my office door. Walking past and working under that gaze is part of being in the tradition.
[5] See Frank's (2000) account of 'the standpoint of storyteller'.

home-centred). The narrative, the painting and the photograph together convey the strength, and the fragility, of persons in relationship in community.

Annie's story articulates the 'ends and goods' of *psychiatric nursing practice* in the tradition: emotional commitment ('my passionate concern'), participation in community ('my affinity with them') and accountability based on argument ('my quest for knowledge about mental illness and health'). It conveys too the 'ends and goods' of the *scholarly practice*: responding to 'intellectual and academic stimulus provided by colleagues and students'; extending knowledge through research and travel; contributing to 'professional, political and scientific progress'.

Annie's story is part of the larger story of the tradition of the Department. The University of Edinburgh was the first University in the UK to offer education to nurses, and appointed the first Professor of Nursing Studies outside the USA. It is the story of pioneering psychiatric and mental health nursing research, with the first Edinburgh PhD in this field awarded in 1960. This body of research comprises an 'historically extended' and 'socially embodied' critique of psychiatric and mental health nursing practice in the local area as it has evolved since the late 1950s. The larger story is that of a 'socially embodied' argument about practice. Research and teaching done by members of the Department challenged this local practice, through critical accounts of the nurse's role (in changing institutions), knowledge base and ethical stance. I will turn now to consider how the tradition became institutionalised in the University.

The University of Edinburgh: context for the tradition

The Nursing Teaching Unit[6] was founded in 1956, originally in the Faculty of Arts. It 'evolved' to become the Department of Nursing Studies in the Faculty of Social Science in 1962/1963 (Weir 1996).

The two figures whose parts in the founding I summarise here, Elsie Stephenson and John Macmurray, were both 'mavericks' (Allan 1990: 108; Costello 2002) who nonetheless were able to use the processes of a powerful university to realise their aim of development of persons through education.

The appointment of Stephenson as founding Director shocked many in the Scottish nursing establishment, as she 'was neither a graduate nor an experienced nurse-educator' (Weir 1996, pp. 12–13). Stephenson brought to the new Unit substantial experience and commitment to the values base of public health nursing. ' "I like the idea of a healthy nation, a healthy world – not purely physical, but in spirit, in body and in mind," she told health visitors . . . in June, 1962 . . .' (Allan 1990: 156). Her view of nursing – 'a listener, a doer, someone who tries to understand the physical, mental and spiritual needs of man from infancy to old age' (Allan 1990: 16) – was consistent with that conveyed in Annie's emblematic story:

---

[6] This then became the Nursing Studies Unit, which became the Department of Nursing Studies.

Elsie's message was clear: there was nothing mysterious about good nursing practice; it demanded simply the combination of compassion for other human beings with the application of sound knowledge of health matters. (Allan 1990: v)

So too was her emphasis on the importance of personal relationships in nursing education.[7] Stephenson set nursing in a social context (seeing it as enabling the person to play his or her part in the community) and legitimated nursing's location in the University accordingly:

Elsie saw nursing as an art and science designed to help the individual retain his rightful place in society, and to teach him how to improve his contribution to, and enjoyment of, the community in which he lived. Nursing seen in this light fitted well into Edinburgh's gigantic Arts Faculty. (Allan 1990: 109)

Stephenson's vision chimed with that of Macmurray, Professor of Moral Philosophy and Dean of the Faculty of Arts when the Nursing Studies Unit was established. In a biography of Macmurray, Costello wrote:

Close to [Macmurray's] heart as Dean [of the Faculty of Arts] was the new Department of Nursing [*sic* – it was the Nursing Studies Unit at that time] which he strove to keep associated with the Arts rather than the Science faculty on the grounds that it is primarily persons that nurses attend to, not diseases. He was convinced, partly from his experience for two years in the Medical Corps in World War I, that healing requires a felt knowledge of the needs of the whole person. His success . . . in achieving that goal in March 1956 was perhaps his most obvious accomplishment in his efforts to maintain the humanistic focus in the University. (Costello 2002: 336)

Macmurray's emphases on nurses 'attending to' persons and on a 'felt knowledge of the needs of the whole person' accord with Annie's views as sketched in the emblematic story. Annie's 'quest for knowledge' (epistemology) and her commitment to and affinity with suffering others (ethics) were consistent with Macmurray's project and 'efforts to maintain the humanistic focus of the University'.

Macmurray's emphasis on 'care for the individual person in his or her individuality' should be noted:

Only care for both the individual person in his or her individuality and for the gathering of free persons in a shared life of meanings and values can create the form of society that Macmurray refers to as 'community.' (Costello 2002: 328)

'Genuinely heterocentric care, affection and respect' (Costello 2002: 13) – relating to the other as *fully* other – were key values in Macmurray's philosophy; and

---

[7] Stephenson's biographer, Sheila Allan, recalled 'the uniquely personal relationship between staff and students in this Department, a tradition which Elsie has firmly established' (Allan 1990: vi).

a premiss for 'the gathering of free persons in a shared life . . . as "community" '. There was thus in Edinburgh a *vision* of how nursing accorded with the structure of the institution, and with the *ideal* of the humanistic university; and a *will* to keep it 'associated with the Arts rather than the Science faculty'.[8] There was *potential* for it to help 'maintain the humanistic focus' by formation (through education) of whole persons, in relationship in community; to be both beneficiary of its situation in the humanistic university and contributor to it through development of knowledge of healing whole persons.

The aims of developing persons and of maintaining the humanistic focus of the University were related, and both required *effort*. However, at the very time that nursing became part of the Arts Faculty, Macmurray's 'fighting for the humanities' was coming to an end (Costello 2002: 307). He retired with a sense that 'the primary place of the humanities has been lost in the passing of a culture' (Costello 2002: 338). Thus from the beginning the 'line' spliced from Stephenson's commitment to the values of whole-person public health nursing (cf. Macmurray 1964) and Macmurray's commitment to values of the humanistic university and the place therein of whole-person nursing, was fragile.

Teaching, supervision and research in the Department

I will now sketch the Department's tradition of teaching, supervision and research on psychiatric nursing in hospital and community as an 'historically extended, socially embodied argument' (MacIntyre 1985: 222). I want to convey a sense of the relationships of influence, support and development between those working in the Department and students doing undergraduate and taught MSc courses, and doing dissertations for higher degrees, whereby *challenge* and *argument* as constitutive goods in this tradition have been 'socially embodied'.

Teaching

The present practices of teaching in the School can be directly linked to practices of those earlier in the tradition; the transmission of knowledge based in part on direct personal influence. One key point to note is that for most of the Department's life teaching on nursing and people with mental illness or mental health problems has been to undergraduates preparing to be general nurses. Until 1988 the Department did not offer a course leading to mental nurse registration. Till then, students had placements in psychiatric settings as part of their general nursing course, and were supervised there by experienced mental health nurses in the Department (e.g. Annie, Ruth Schrock, Susan Sladden). These people contributed to teaching on social scientific aspects of health and illness (individuality, person,

---

[8] We see here prefigured Desmond Ryan's argument that nursing is one of the 'person arts' (Ryan 1985).

family and community). They also had specific sessions geared to the students' periods of experience in psychiatric settings in which they aimed to enable students to relate both 'theory' and what they encountered in practice settings to their own experiences of, e.g., aggression or irrationality. The focus was on making experiences in practice settings meaningful from the students' own perspectives, and relating this learning also to their experience and learning in other areas of nursing.[9] This teaching can be considered as contributing to the Department's distinctive education of nurses for holistic or 'whole-person' practice in a social science disciplinary context (see above on Stephenson; and below on John's research). During this period, while the students pursuing general nurse registration would have known of the psychiatric nursing backgrounds of these teachers, they would have seen them mainly as teachers. These teachers' thinking was influenced by a notion of therapeutic community 'in the widest sense', informed by an 'ideology of democracy, equality and empowerment' (Ruth Schrock, personal communication).[10,11]

Influenced by their placements, the teaching and the teachers as role models, some of these students became interested in psychiatric nursing and wanted to train and work in that field. However, until the Mental Health Branch started in 1988, students in the Department who wanted to qualify as mental nurses had to go elsewhere to do so after graduating as general nurses. Examples of those who did so include nurses who later made substantial contributions to psychiatric nursing practice and research (e.g. Sarah Whicher, Sue Simmons and Linda Pollock).

Anne Robertson, who was an undergraduate in the Department in the 1980s and is now the lecturer with main responsibility for the mental health branch programme, followed that path. She had found Annie an inspirational teacher. For example, in a group tutorial Annie had asked the class something and there was silence. Silence, and discomfort. Annie said: 'Perhaps I should open a window and let the air circulate – nothing else is moving here!' Other students looked uncomfortable but Anne laughed, en route to deciding she wanted to learn how to teach like Annie.[12] Anne went to the Maudsley for her mental health nurse

---

[9] In doing this Annie would have drawn on her Maudsley teaching experience and on her visit to the USA in 1960–61. In part, at least, her motivation for that trip stemmed from grappling with the problem of teaching general nursing students doing short placements at the Maudsley. American texts, especially Greenblatt *et al.* (1955), indicated that answers to those problems might be found in the USA.

[10] Anne Robertson says she saw Annie as an inspirational educationalist, not as a psychiatric nurse.

[11] I am indebted to Ruth Schrock, Susan Sladden and Anne Robertson for conversations on the Department's teaching relating to mental health and illness in this period.

[12] Another colleague said that when she and a classmate met for a reunion recently, the first thing they reminisced about was their class in nursing at the University, on understanding of normal health. Annie was the teacher. She sat facing the class and asked 'What is normal?' The students sat, waiting. They looked at her but she said nothing. They looked at their notebooks, at each other, around. Then Annie said: 'Look at me!' They looked. 'What is normal?' My colleague described Annie as she saw and heard her – body shape, glasses, accent. All this the students remembered.

training, subsequently returning to Edinburgh to work at the Royal Edinburgh Hospital. She joined the Department in 1988 to develop the curriculum on mental health for the overall undergraduate programme, and specifically to develop the new integrated BSc degree and RMN (Registered Mental Nurse) programme. She built on earlier teaching in the Department (e.g. Rosemary Weir's involvement of students in curriculum construction) and on a pedagogy emphasising experiential learning, reflection and group work (the latter drawing on knowledge gained at the Maudsley from her teacher there, Gunna Dietrich). Anne thus continued the tradition of links between the Maudsley and the Department.

The practice of requiring and challenging others to give an account of what they thought or did was fundamental to Annie's teaching.[13] It was central to the tradition of therapeutic community work with which she had been involved at Mill Hill and at the Maudsley. In addition, Annie had visited the USA in 1960–1961 and gained first-hand knowledge of American psychiatric nursing practice and education (Altschul 1960:2001a, b, 1961:2001a, b). There she became disillusioned with the nursing practice and nursing education she observed:

> It seemed . . . that the intensive one-to-one relationship had little bearing on the practice of psychiatric nursing as it occurred on the ward. (Altschul 1972: 5)

She criticised what she saw as *unquestioning* acceptance of the ideology of the one-to-one relationship. It jarred with her commitment to question and argue about practice and education and to require others to do likewise, and with her commitment to responding to the patient in his or her social context.

Annie's conception of psychiatric nursing when she joined the Department in 1964, and an indication of its congruence with the values of Stephenson and Macmurray, are seen in a text from that year:

> Psychiatric nursing is concerned with the promotion of mental health, the prevention of mental disorder and the nursing care of patients with mental illness . . . Mental health . . . which has been defined as 'the full and harmonious functioning of the whole personality', can best be studied by reference to mental illness. The nurse is seeking to promote the mental health and happiness of her patients. (Altschul 1964: 3)

Perhaps as important as Annie's fit with the receiving academic context was her fit with the local clinical context. Henry Walton (now Emeritus Professor of Psychiatry and International Medical Education at the University of Edinburgh), a former colleague of Annie's at the Maudsley, had recently come to Edinburgh to develop a therapeutic community context at the Royal Edinburgh Hospital. He had encouraged Annie to apply for the World Health Organization-funded

---

[13] It was characteristic of practice at the Maudsley Hospital, too, when Anne Robertson did her mental health training there after graduation from this University.

lectureship in the Nursing Studies Unit because he saw 'the educational necessity of establishing, as an essential component, the concept of the autonomous, self-directed nurse as a key member of the therapeutic team' (Henry Walton, personal communication). According to Walton, the Royal Edinburgh Hospital was Annie's informal clinical base following her appointment at the University:

> Annie, with enthusiasm and educational zeal, came and began her huge participation in the local renewal of psychiatry, leading in time to the wry, widespread acknowledgment that a MacMaudsley had been established in Scotland. (Henry Walton, personal communication; see also Tilley 2002)

Walton notes too the wider range of Annie's contributions while a member of the Department, her extensive World Health Organization work 'an aspect of her professional persona greatly valued internationally' (Henry Walton, personal communication).

Walton elaborated the virtues of 'autonomous, self-directed practice' in the therapeutic community context. The person was 'on view, open to inspection' in such a way that others could 'see for themselves, and make their own judgements' about the other's practice. This openness to 'general inspection' meant the person was 'laying [her or his] self on the line' (Henry Walton, personal communication).[14]

In our current teaching of undergraduates (common foundation course and mental health branch students) Anne Robertson and I aim to realise a number of goods and practices. These include: openness to criticism; resistance to ideology; and autonomous, self-directed practice as part of a collective effort to restore the person experiencing mental distress or illness to health and participation in community. If these goods sound 'airy', the ways in which they were realised are not. The practice of psychiatric nursing, for Annie, was grounded in knowing and 'doing alongside' the patient:

> I would summarise what psychiatric nurses do thus: they try to get to know their patient. They do it mostly by listening and observing . . . Getting to know the patient cannot be

---

[14] This therapeutic community tradition, which Annie brought to Edinburgh, can also be discerned in an account she gave of 'learning objectives for clinical practice':

- those which relate to the creation of a therapeutic environment;
- those which concern observation, interpretation and reporting of observations;
- communication with a patient, one-to-one, listening, forming a relationship, monitoring the effect of this on the patient and the nurse; and
- communicating with patients in a group setting and dealing with relationships between members of the group. (Altschul 1997: 11)

See page 47, this chapter, regarding Annie's view of American practice.

hurried. Knowledge of people develops incrementally, sometimes in the process of observation and listening alone, but more commonly in the process of doing things together, working, playing, eating, learning, drinking coffee together and smoking. Psychiatric nurses do, alongside the patients, all the things people normally do in their lives. They look after their physical well-being, socialise, indulge in leisure activities, work, shop, garden, clean their homes, decorate, go for walks, spend money, argue, read, study, eat and form relationships. (Altschul 1997: 8)

This is a fair account of what our students do in practice with people in various settings.

The challenge motivating us is to enable each student to embark on his or her *own* quest for understanding of the question *'Call yourself a nurse?'* and the student's own and others' answers. We aim to enable students to appraise critically the radically different understandings of mental health and illness now current in the field. We want our students to be able to negotiate current discourse shifts, to engage with people – health service workers, service users and survivors – in settings in which their senses of self and other, relationship and community, are structured by sometimes conflicting discourses. As they 'do alongside' people/patients, move between institutions and work across discourses, we want them to hold themselves and the institutions to account.

Practise of argument, based on a model of the nurse as rhetorician (Tilley 1997) is specifically institutionalised in our curriculum in a course on research methods for undergraduates and in a Masters course on Debates and Developments in Mental Health Care. In teaching these topics, using these methods, we aim to enable each student to learn to practise according to the 'perennial ethic' (Smith 1982). This entails obligations: to practise and argue congruently with the student's own values, seeing him/herself as fully one; to attend carefully to the values and arguments of the other, seeing the other as fully one; and to accept the better argument.[15] We want our students to accept the responsibilities of principled heterocentrism, resisting hegemonic discourses and creating possibilities for free participation in the community.

Our ability to see each student in this way is no doubt enhanced by the small numbers of students who follow the mental health branch. Some years we do not have enough students wanting to do the mental health branch to be able to offer the course. Three staff are required to sustain the course, and we ourselves have to argue the case for keeping this variety of educational practice alive.

---

[15] In a paper titled *Sustaining Varieties of Practice* (Tilley, 1998), I identified features of the then-topical dispute between two key figures in the field, Prof Kevin Gournay and Prof Phil Barker; and considered whether implicit in the position of each (as characterised) there were grounds for a better argument. I did this under the auspice of the good of sustaining variety of practice (and of argument about and within practice). Prof Gournay and Prof Barker were seen as two persons in relationship (of argument capable of development) in a 'community' (of others in the fields of practice and academic nursing).

Supervision

Supervision of dissertations – Honours, taught Masters and higher degrees by research – is the second 'historically extended, socially embodied' practice central to the tradition. The supervision relationship is a key site and vehicle for transmission of the values and practices of the tradition. I have supervised three of the authors of chapters in this book at one level or another. Former mental health undergraduates and masters students have published papers based on their dissertations supervised by Anne or myself.

The longest-established and most distinctive element is supervision of dissertations written for higher degrees (MPhil or PhD); a number of which were subsequently published as monographs. Based on studies done in local hospitals or community settings, the dissertations are key documents of a *local* tradition of psychiatric nursing research. Taken together they record an extended, intertextual argument, by a succession of scholars, about the adequacy of psychiatric practitioners' accounts of practice, and also about the adequacy of the accounts produced by other scholars in the tradition. The products of this local tradition in an emerging field were influential in representing, and constructing, the field of Scottish or UK mental health nursing (Tilley 1997).

These texts, written for higher degrees and subsequently published, constitute Edinburgh's unique contribution to (construction of) the field of knowledge of psychiatric and mental health nursing. Supervision, or related support from others in the tradition, has been vital to this work. Audrey John, a general nurse whose 1960 dissertation on acute wards in mental hospitals was the first in the line, acknowledged the support of Elsie Stephenson. Annie Altschul was supervised by Elsie Stephenson and by Henry Walton. Annie supervised Ruth Schrock (a psychiatric nurse whose dissertation was on philosophy and nursing) and Alison Tierney (whose dissertation was on people with learning difficulties). Ruth Schrock supervised Susan Sladden who supervised Linda Pollock, Maxine Mueller and me. I supervised Sue Cowan, Susanne Forrest, Martin Gaughan and Paul Currie. Penny Prophit[16] supervised Eamon Shanley and Gordon Turner.[17] See Fig. 3.1 for titles of dissertations by students who have done mental-health-related dissertations.

The qualities of the process of supervision are conveyed through acknowledgements in the dissertations, and through stories. For example, in her acknowledgements, Ruth Schrock cited:

---

[16] Penny Prophit, Professor of Nursing Studies in the Department from 1983–1992, had a psychiatric nursing background. She contributed to teaching on development and on stress and burnout, as well as on nursing knowledge.

[17] Each student had a second supervisor who may have been as significant as – or more significant than – these I have mentioned.

Year	Name	MSc (Social Science) Thesis Title	Nursing Studies Supervisor
1967	ALTSCHUL Annie	Measurement of patient–nurse interaction in relation to in-patient psychiatric treatment	STEPHENSON Elsie

Year	Name	MPhil Thesis Title	Nursing Studies Supervisor/s
1998	GAUGHAN Martin	An evaluation of a day programme for young people with psychiatric/ emotional problems (perspectives from users and providers)	TILLEY Stephen
1997	CURRIE Paul	A study of hospital and voluntary mental health service usage by the Asian and Chinese communities in Edinburgh	TILLEY Stephen
1992	FORREST Susanne	Hospital and community: clients' and carers' experience of life in two residential settings for the mentally ill	TILLEY Stephen
1981	SUGDEN J.M.	Nursing activity and some variables in the psychiatric treatment process	ALTSCHUL Annie

Year	Name	PhD Thesis Title	Nursing Studies Supervisor/s
1997	COWAN Susan	Views on community care for people with mental health problems: a discourse analysis of argument and accountability in a Scottish community	TILLEY Stephen
1995	MUELLER Maxine	Organising participation: an ethnography of 'community' in hospital	SLADDEN Susan
1994	TURNER Gordon	Organisational climate and standards of nursing care: the administration of depot neuroleptic drugs to psychiatric out-patients	ATKINSON, Ian PROPHIT, Penny MELIA, Kath

Fig. 3.1 Higher degrees by research at the University of Edinburgh: psychiatric and mental health nursing.

1990	TILLEY Stephen	Negotiating realities: making sense of interaction between patients diagnosed as neurotic and nurses in two psychiatric admission wards	SLADDEN Susan
1988	POLLOCK Linda	Community psychiatric nursing explained: an analysis of the views of patients, carers and nurses	SLADDEN Susan
1984	SHANLEY J.E.R.	Evaluation of mental nurses by their patients and charge nurses	ALTSCHUL, Annie DAVIS, Bryn PROPHIT, Penny
1981	SCHRÖCK Ruth	An argument concerning the meaning and relevance of philosophical enquiries in nursing	ALTSCHUL Annie
1977	SLADDEN S.	Psychiatric community nursing: a study of a working situation	SCHRÖCK Ruth
1959	JOHN A.L.	A study of the psychiatric nurse and his/her role in the care of the mentally ill	No record of supervisor's name could be found

Fig. 3.1 *(cont'd)*

Annie Altschul, professor of nursing at the University of Edinburgh, who as teacher, colleague and supervisor has contributed more than anyone to help me think as clearly as I can and who has shown continued patience in the face of both procrastination and panic. (Schrock 1981)

A dedication by John in the front of a copy of the monograph based on her dissertation reads:

Elsie – With grateful thanks for all the opportunities, and the encouragement & support which lies behind the finished product. Audrey. 11th May 1961.

According to one former student, supervision by Annie generated negative as well as positive feelings. Two aspects of supervision stood out for this person: Annie addressing the dilemmatic desires for completion and perfection: and her maxim 'It's the student's thesis, not the supervisor's'.

As with teaching, supervision in the tradition is an institutionally supported vehicle for development of the person/scholar through relationship in a form of community. This element of the tradition too is now fragile, subject to some strain as the ratio of postgraduate research students to staff increases.

Research

Since the late 1950s figures in the tradition have carried out research on psychiatric and mental health nursing, mainly in the local area (Edinburgh, Lothian and the adjacent counties or regions). Some of this research has been done without funding, some with small- to medium-scale funding (e.g. MacDonald & Altschul 1972; Tilley & Pollock 2001). The main form in which research has been institutionalised in the Department has been the succession of dissertations done for higher degrees. Some of this research has been carried out as part of funded projects; some has been supported by Scottish Office research training studentships held by students housed in the Department's Nursing Research Unit (funded by the Scottish Office from 1971–1994).

Research is one of the main ways in which those in the tradition challenged both psychiatric and mental health nurses and other scholars. Typically through qualitative studies, entailing formation of research-related relationships with practitioners and patients, they challenge psychiatric and mental health nurses to account for their practice. They interpret those practitioners' accounts in professional, policy and institutional contexts, explicitly or implicitly evaluating practice and proposing changes. A central theme is their interpretation and evaluation of the nurses and patients as persons in relationship in community.

The researchers also challenge other researchers in the tradition, and outside it, regarding the adequacy of the other researchers' accounts, e.g. of methods. For example, Ruth Schrock's dissertation, while not focused on mental health, can be seen in this light; challenging nursing theorists, students and practitioners to step back and consider epistemological issues in the development of knowledge for nursing:

> In the search for nursing knowledge for practical, professional, academic and personal purposes, criteria for its identification need to be developed (Schrock, 1981, Abstract). It is only through the integrated efforts of the philosopher, the historian, the empirical scientist and the professional practitioner that nursing knowledge can be gained, developed and advanced, and the discipline of nursing be created. (Schrock 1981: 302)

To substantiate these claims I will focus on arguments made by five people who completed their higher degrees at the University and were also members of the Department teaching or research staff, or connected to the Department through a partnership with the local trust.

(1) *Audrey John*. John was a Rockefeller Research Fellow in the Nursing Studies Unit (Weir 1996). Her PhD thesis (John 1960) was published as the monograph *A Study of the Psychiatric Nurse* (John 1961). She set her study of the 'working situation' of nurses in admission wards in four mental hospitals in the context of contemporary public awareness of 'the outstanding burden of mental illness in the community and of its significance' (p. 1) and social science critiques of the mental hospital. She aimed to investigate 'whether

psychiatric nursing is fundamentally different from any other type of good nursing care' and 'the nurse's relationship with her patients' (p. 3).

John challenged the practice she observed, in terms that reflect her professional values base, and then-contemporary policy and social contexts. 'Psychiatrically, the mental health nurse has been called upon to change *fundamental* attitudes to patient-care' (p. 40, italics in original); however, 'too little nursing attention of both a psychological and physical nature was available . . . to achieve the complete transition from custodial to therapeutic care' (p. 100). This represented a failure to achieve changes in nurse–patient relationships despite the 'spirit' of the then-new Mental Health Act, 1959:

> The unlocking of doors, whilst relaxing general ward tension, has undoubtedly multiplied the responsibilities of the nurse towards her patients. The spiritual, intellectual and social aspects of their personalities, which at one time it might have been possible to ignore, are beginning to take their rightful place in treatment of the patient as a 'whole person'. With increased understanding of patient needs, has also come the charge to meet those needs as adequately as possible . . . Without adequate knowledge of her patients she cannot hope to fulfil her function efficiently. (p. 41)

Such 'whole person' relationships (which would have fulfilled some of Stephenson's and Macmurray's ambitions for nursing) were not evident. Instead, the nurses' work was more 'custodial' than 'professional' and 'therapeutic'; characterised by 'a loss of "vocation" in the work, infiltration of a "lay" attitude' and 'identification with the general community' (pp. 116–117), and routine that 'discouraged [the nurses from] thinking' (p. 140). To remedy this, John proposed clarification of the 'function (and status) of the qualified psychiatric nurse' (p. 151) and a 'comprehensive basic training . . . the logical conclusion to the acknowledgement of the patient as a whole person' (p. 153). (The subsequent tradition of teaching in the Department, described above, went some way towards achieving this.) In John's text, 'community' (source of lay attitudes) is inimical to the therapeutic function of the hospital; as is the stultifying dullness of the custodial role. The development of the 'whole person' is to be achieved by development of a more professional values and knowledge base.

(2) *Annie Altschul.* Annie challenged practice on the grounds that it was not theoretically grounded, not reflexive and not open to questioning. The challenge was grounded in her practice experience (especially in therapeutic communities), her wide knowledge of the field and well-honed critical faculties.

In the study she did for her MSc (Social Science) degree at Edinburgh [Altschul 1967; published as the influential monograph *Patient-Nurse Interaction* (Altschul 1972)] Annie continued her 'quest for knowledge about mental illness'. Prior to her visit to the USA in 1960–1961, Annie had read a text (Greenblatt *et al.* 1955) that characterised 'nursing therapy' [devised by June Mellow (Mellow 1964) and based on the one-to-one relationship] as a key element in the change 'from custodial to therapeutic attitudes' in the hospital.

She was, however, disillusioned with the practice and nursing education she observed on her US visit. She saw American nurses as unwilling to argue about practice, and accepting unquestioningly the ideology of the one-to-one relationship; telling Mellow, her teacher and supervisor in Boston, that Greenblatt *et al.* had 'render(ed) reality unrecognizable' (Altschul 1960:2001b: 66), (mis)representing the reality of practice and the patient's experience.

Annie's US visit 'started a train of thought which I shall pursue for some time to come, namely to determine what really are the theoretical foundations on which psychiatric nursing is based' (Altschul 1961:2001b). For the Altschul paper and related commentaries on her 1960–61 visit, http://www.qmuc.ac.lkl/hn/history/AnnieA/index.html, Tilley, S. with Mortimer, B. (eds) A Festschrift for Professor Annie Altschul. Her MSc dissertation can be read as an attempt to do this.[18] To remedy the 'one-sided approach to the study of nurse–patient relationship', and due to the complexity of studying relationships directly, she carried out an observational study of dyadic interaction, followed by interviews in which she asked nurses to account for their role in the interaction. She also asked those nurses and patients whom she surmised to have 'special relationships' about those relationships.

Her findings echo those of John (a frequent reference)[19]. I have discussed Annie's study in detail elsewhere (Tilley 1995, 1999b) and here note only that she critiqued nurses for

- inadequacies in their thinking about and accounting for practice (which she saw as based on a 'general "common sense" approach', indistinguishable from that of 'lay' people);
- limited therapeutic effect [their relationships with patients 'experienced as therapeutic by the patients concerned' (p. 192) but unlikely to be therapeutic judged by criteria set by American nursing theorists (p. 190)].

She proposed a remedy based on reconfiguring the nurse's accountability:

> If nurses were asked to account for their interactions, junior nurses by senior nurses, and all nurses by doctors, if senior nurses were asked to make more explicit what at present is being done without insight, a great deal of existing skill would become observable, and some lack of skill would be remedied. There seems to be an urgent need for a deliberate and conscious effort to increase communications and to increase observability of patients by nurses, of nurses by each other, and between nurses and doctors. Only then can the necessary theoretical background for effective interaction with patients become available. (Altschul 1972: 196)

---

[18] Ruth Schröck says that the ideology of the one-to-one relationship was at that time also being promoted in Scotland, with Annie a skeptic, saying that there was no empirical evidence to support claims for this form of practice, and that one could not talk about the relationship until one knew what *contact* the nurse had with the patient (Ruth Schrock, personal communication).

[19] John was a frequent reference, and the main British psychiatric nursing reference, in Annie's seminal text *Patient–Nurse Interaction*, based on her Edinburgh MSc (Social Science) thesis.

Annie's challenge to Scottish nurses in the institution which Walton described as her 'informal clinical base' should be read in light of her earlier challenge to June Mellow and colleagues in Boston. The proposed system of accounting would develop in local practice settings something missing in Boston: the questioning of practice which formed such an essential component of therapeutic community work.[20,21] That change in practice would develop the theoretical basis of practice and nurses' capacity to form therapeutic relationships. The development of the nurse as professional (and of the patient through a more therapeutic relationship with the nurse) would be achieved through development of inter-professional communication in a quasi-therapeutic community environment.

(3) *Susan Sladden.* Sladden acknowledged her 'debt to the influence and active help of Professor Annie Altschul' [Sladden 1979, third (unnumbered) page in Preface]. She had trained in psychiatric nursing at Dingleton Hospital [resisting pressures to commit wholly to the therapeutic community ideology (Susan Sladden, personal communication)]. She also 'spliced' into the Department her experience both of nursing practice and knowledge of social policy based on earlier work in the civil service and study for a Diploma in Social Administration.

Sladden's PhD thesis (Sladden 1977) was later published as *Psychiatric Nursing in the Community: A Study of a Working Situation* (Sladden 1979). She conceived her study as 'a contribution to a more satisfactory definition of the psychiatric nurse's role in the community' (p. 52), intended to develop a 'model' of community psychiatric nursing care' (p. 58).

Sladden both drew on and critiqued the work of John and Altschul. She cited both on 'inadequate definition of the psychiatric nurse's role, and other disparities between nursing roles as prescribed and nurses' observed role performance' (p. 31). She followed both in highlighting the importance of the nurse–patient relationship (e.g. finding evidence of beneficial flexibility in community psychiatric nurses' (CPNs) work with people with longer-term illnesses who also had difficulties in forming relationships). She built

---

[20] Altschul carried out or held the grant for two studies of community psychiatric nursing at Dingleton Hospital (Altschul 1973, 1983). Maxwell Jones, with whom Annie had worked in London, had established Dingleton as the leading example of therapeutic community orientation in a Scottish hospital.
[21] Annie distinguished 'learning objectives for clinical practice' as she saw them (see footnote 14) from those she found during a visit to the USA in 1960–1961:

My experience in the USA showed that emphasis was placed mainly on [learning] to form and maintain a relationship with one patient and, in weekly sessions with their mentor, [learning] how to use this in a therapeutic way . . . My view is that this aspect of the psychiatric nurse's function is only one part of her/his function, and that for many patients it is not the most important one. Sharing the patient's daily life, wherever that may be, observing and communicating in the course of other activities, piecing together a picture of the patient from fragments of information obtained as a by-product of activities, is in my opinion every bit as important. (Altschul 1997: 11)

on the methodological work Annie had done in two studies of community psychiatric nursing at Dingleton Hospital[22] but demurred from some of Annie's conclusions, e.g. that it was 'useless' to teach nurses interactional skills since they thought these 'intuitive' (p. 181).

Sladden analysed the 'ambiguities and problems' of psychiatric nursing. Whereas John had construed these in terms of nursing professionalisation, and Annie in terms of a lack of theoretical basis and communication about practice, Sladden situated them at a different level in the social system:

> Psychiatric nursing shares many of the current ambiguities and problems in understanding the function of psychiatry in society. It is not at all clear whether the two fundamentally different roles which have emerged – that of a psychosocial therapist and that of an auxiliary worker in a branch of medicine – can be reconciled in one person or whether they will prove to be incompatible.' (p. 40)

> 'The major source of ambiguity and inconsistency seemed to lie in a failure to relate the service and its objectives to a consistent model of what community care should mean in the context of psychiatry. (p. 178)

Thus Sladden contextualised the problems of accounting for the psychiatric nurse's role ('worker in a complex situation') in a policy and historical context. She thought it unwise to try to specify too closely the elements of the CPN's role, suggesting as a 'guiding principle [for] . . . psychiatric services' the 'capacity for flexible adaptation to the needs of patients' (p. 180). She nonetheless critiqued CPNs' failure to make clear the 'ideologies' on which they based their relationships with patients in the community. She thought that research should inform values-based judgement[23], and proposed: 'If there is one lesson to be learned from this study, it is the need for those who work in the same field to agree about the nature and purpose of the task at hand' (p. 183).

(4) *Linda Pollock.* Pollock, in her PhD thesis [(Pollock 1988); published as *Community Psychiatric Nursing: Myth and Reality* (Pollock 1989)], saw the development of community psychiatric nursing as 'local in nature' and so justified her study being done at the 'local level' (p. 65), with CPN teams in two hospitals. Her study was 'motivated by the concern to examine critically the work of community psychiatric nurses' to 'provide a sound foundation for development'.

She cited Annie's Dingleton studies as 'exemplary', noting Annie's methodological response to 'nurses' difficulty in talking in detail about their thoughts, feelings, perceptions and actions' (p. 82). Pollock's own methodological

---

[22] Sladden cited Annie's finding (Altschul 1973) that 'evidence of different use of professional skills was not obtained. On the contrary, the hospital culture, emphasizing similarities of function . . . was maintained' (Sladden, 1979, p. 46). While this aspect of the therapeutic community tradition was maintained when nurses started working in the natural community, other aspects were not.

[23] 'Where matters of value and expediency are in question, facts – however reliable and valid – are no substitute for the exercise of judgement. Research . . . may . . . provide a starting point for discussion of the objectives and values on which decisions should be based.' (Sladden, 1979, p. 5)

contributions shed light on the problem of nurses' failure to conceptualise (a theme in John's, Altschul's and Sladden's work). Through use of a repertory grid method which 'made respondents think' (p. 191), Pollock developed the argument among researchers in the tradition about practising nurses' limitations as accountable practitioners. Her account of the accountable nurse is qualitatively different from John's and from Altschul's (the nurse who did not think, and the nurse without a theoretical background).

Similarly, her analysis provided a picture of the nurses' role in making community care 'work':

> The community psychiatric nurses can be likened to the characters in a play whose title is 'The provision of a community psychiatric nursing service', the plot being the provision of individualised care. (p. 115)

A quarter of a century earlier Annie had challenged June Mellow and her Boston academic colleagues for 'render(ing) the reality [of hospital life as experienced] unrecognisable'. Pollock found that CPNs obscured the 'reality' of scarce resources, the nurses being 'obliged' to 'make compromises' 'in order to make the ideology [of "individualised care"] fit the resources' (p. 193). Pollock thus challenged the CPNs for being insufficiently critical of the consequences of their taking on the 'obligation' to 'make the system work'. The plot of the 'play' is ironic: the nurses' self-claimed 'patient-focused' work (p. 116) and 'emphasis [on] developing relationships' (p. 186) sustained a service that did not provide 'individualised care' (p. 193). Sensitive to the implications of this charge, Pollock proposed a dual strategy to help CPNs in this predicament: training focused both on 'skills acquisition' and on 'moral philosophy' (p. 203).

(5) *Tilley.* My doctoral dissertation [(Tilley 1990), later published as *Negotiating Realities* (Tilley 1995)] was based on an interpretive study of interaction between patients diagnosed as neurotic and nurses in two Scottish psychiatric admission wards. In it I challenged previous research – including some in this tradition – which had called into question nurses' knowledge (common sense versus theoretical knowledge), effectiveness and moral stance in relation to these patients. Using an 'accounts' methodology, I found that through their conversation these nurses and patients constructed knowledge, negotiated relations of power and maintained and repaired moral orders. Their interaction was situated in, and reflexively maintained, the wards as sites of assessment and treatment. I used Berger and Luckmann's concepts of social construction of reality and 'therapy' to interpret their interaction as remedy for the patients' departures from common sense. The concept of common sense was indispensable for understanding how nurses and patients managed their interaction and their accounts.

I challenged what I saw as limitations of Annie's method and argument in *Patient–Nurse Interaction*. For example, she found that nurses accounted to her for what they had done in interaction by invoking 'common sense'.

Annie argued that 'common sense' could not be the basis for action, given that nurses had done what she regarded as different things with the same patient in the same situation (see Tilley 1995, 1999b). I argued that in doing so she had failed to acknowledge the implications of her *own* use of common sense. I further argued that the nurses' use of common sense as resource in appraising the adequacy of patients' accounts was an essential aspect of their work in recovering 'strays' from the 'paramount reality' of everyday life, and restoring them to the community, the shared life-space, ordered by common sense. Common sense, not theoretical commitment, was the fundamental basis for relationship of persons in community.[24]

Annie was the internal examiner for my PhD. She did not challenge my argument on that occasion; but did, subsequently, writing 'I am not against common sense. But my job was to teach students, and common sense is not something that can be taught' (Altschul 1999). In writing thus, Annie was not (as I had construed her in my thesis) standing *outside* the situation of practice, holding up a template of theoretical knowledge and noting only 'absence'. Rather, she was speaking from her fundamental standpoint as *teacher*[25,26], articulating the epistemological and ethical base from which she addressed and constituted her community. From her perspective, if common sense were sufficient, she could not practise accountably as a teacher. Annie as *researcher* was acting accountably as the nurse *teacher* asking questions of – challenging – practitioners. That she did not challenge them *in* the research setting to elucidate the problematic of common sense in that situation remains, I think, methodologically problematic. Nonetheless, I now see her as having acted accountably in asking the *other* (in the research situation, the nurse in practice; in the later argument about argument, myself) to account for his or her practice. In doing so she was practising the virtues of the therapeutic community in research, as she had in practice as a nurse and as a teacher. As teacher, she could not let the nurse (or me) rest with the implication of failure to offer an account 'beyond' 'it's common sense'.[27] Splicing my argument with Annie's (and John's, and Sladden's and Pollock's) I took, and take, my place in the tradition and in mental health nursing.

---

[24] This view is consistent with findings from Altschul, Sladden and Pollock that patients/persons value their work with nurses, albeit that work was found to be insufficiently theoretically informed.

[25] On 'standpoint' see Frank (2000).

[26] On another occasion Annie noted that she had begun a mathematics degree in Vienna before having to leave that city. (Characteristically, much later in life she completed a degree in mathematics.) She said that had she not had to leave Vienna, she probably would have become a maths teacher. 'I don't know what kind of teacher I would have been,' she said, adding with a smile: 'I don't think I would have had trouble in the classroom'. She said that people commented when she was a sister at the Maudsley that the wards were not 'disturbed' when she was on duty (Altschul, in discussion at the *Festschrift for Professor Emeritus Annie Altschul*, Edinburgh, November 2001).

[27] The motivation that had taken her to Boston – to answer the question of how to teach psychiatric nursing, and what to teach, the question with which she returned from Boston – remained live for her.

Sustaining the fragile tradition

In this chapter I have documented the substantial contributions that a small number of psychiatric and mental health nurses have made to research and to development of successive generations of practitioners and research students in the Department. I have portrayed the Department's tradition of challenging general and mental health nurses in educational settings, and psychiatric and mental health nurses in practice settings *reflexively* in order to accomplish three aims. These aims are: (1) to account for and argue about nursing practice in professional, policy and institutional contexts; (2) to change their practices in light of (1); and (3) to appraise reflexively and critically the basis of relationships in practice.

   This tradition is now particularly fragile, in part because we find it increasingly difficult to sustain commitment to these goods at a time of substantial curriculum change, with reduced staff resources. It is also fragile because our institutional context has radically changed, and the institutional story of which we (and the tradition) are a part is being rewritten. In 2002, the Faculties of Arts and of Social Science, along with the rest of the University, were 'restructured', their elements redistributed into new entities (subject areas and Schools in Colleges). We are negotiating where our home will be in the reorganised University,[28] and have been doing so in discussion with colleagues in the College of Medicine, including Community Health Sciences and Public Health, and in the College of Humanities and Social Science. What is 'essential' in our identity, its principled basis, must be preserved in this context. The vision of realising a humanistic university is more fragile even than in Macmurray's day. The various pressures (determination of resources by Research Assessment Exercise results, funding insecurities, pressure to generate income through expansion) that universities now face make it increasingly difficult for us as teachers and supervisors to focus the institution's resources for the benefit and formation of the student/person (cf. Ryan 1985).

   We also have to realise the goods of the tradition in the changing practice, social and cultural contexts in which we find ourselves. In acting as members of the University, as in teaching, supervision and research, we have a responsibility to be free. This responsibility is an implication of principled heterocentrism and commitment to sustaining the possibility of community [see Costello (2002) on Macmurray, above]. In this University as in the higher education sector generally our prospects for fulfilling this responsibility are compromised, our freedoms to teach and research constrained by the demands of corporate accountability and by pressures to increase 'performance' to secure funding. Our ability to tell our own story is in jeopardy. To hold to our responsibility to relate to the other (student/person, patient/person, research participant/person) *as* other we have

---

[28] The Department of Nursing Studies became, for a year, the School of Nursing Studies. Now Nursing Studies is a 'subject area' in the School of Health in Social Science, in the College of Humanities and Social Science.

to defend our own freedom and individuality and fight for the humanistic university as a site for person (not corporate) development.

On this depends our continuing ability to sustain the goods central to our practice and tradition, in our interaction with others in our present practice and policy contexts. An example of that interaction is our partnership with the local Primary Care NHS Trust with responsibilities including community mental health services and the Royal Edinburgh Hospital. Linda Pollock is Nursing Director of that Trust. The partnership offers the potential to realise the goods of tradition through this relationship with practitioners and the community, but only if we hold to our values. Only if we do that can we continue to offer the prospect of development of practitioner/persons, through relationships in the University, contributing to the health of the community we, with others, form through thought and action.[29]

I began with Annie's exemplary narrative. The fragility of the tradition, and its potential, are captured in a more recent 'quest story'. Tessa Parkes, an Honours graduate of our Department, wrote a chapter titled 'My Journey Into, Through and Beyond Psychiatric Nursing' (Parkes 1997) for a book I edited on *The Mental Health Nurse: Views of Practice and Education*. She described being unable to practice the kind of nursing she thought appropriate in the health services settings she came across in her training and thereafter. She encountered people suffering, and she herself suffered when unable to work and to relate to these people in the ways she thought right. She subsequently worked in a voluntary-sector mental health organisation, and then moved into research as an ally with service users, completing a qualitative PhD study at the University of Kent at Canterbury, on the politics of user involvement (Parkes 2002).

In her thesis Tessa revisited her experience while a student in the Department:

> When I entered psychiatric nursing as a student I was completely unprepared for the experience . . . After a few weeks on the ward I began to understand that my initial assumptions about the treatment, care and knowledge underpinning psychiatric practice, were not based on the reality of which I was now a part . . . I grew more and more aware of the disparities between the claims psychiatry was making about its ability to cope with human distress, and the blatant chaos of the everyday reality which I was experiencing . . . I see myself as a survivor of psychiatry, too, though in a different way . . . I left nursing after six months of working as an RMN staff nurse . . . [In a voluntary sector mental health organisation I had an opportunity] to put into practice my ideas of support [which] helped me recover from my experience of front-line nursing and I began to formulate some of the questions I address in this research . . . What makes practice empowering? . . . So reluctantly, after a number of happy and challenging years in [the voluntary agency], I left in order to set about answering these questions. (Parkes 2002: 6)

---

[29] This is consistent with Macmurray's maxim: 'All meaningful thought is for the sake of action, and all meaningful action is for the sake of friendship' (Macmurray 1957: 15). 'The positive form of ["the personal relationship"] goes by many names: love, friendship, fellowship, communion and community . . . [terms] Macmurray used . . . sometimes interchangeably' (Costello 2002: 326).

Tessa's account challenges both the academic institution (the Department) and the psychiatric institutions in which she worked as a student and after qualifying. Her challenge represents the working out of an 'epistemological crisis' (MacIntyre 1989) akin to Annie's in Boston. Annie found that practice as prescribed by texts and teachers was not applied in practice, and did not fit the reality she saw. She asked *'How could I have been so wrong?'* and diagnosed misrepresentation of the practice. Tessa found a mismatch between the possibilities for practice (on the values base of being a person, with the other a person) which she had developed as a student in the Department, and the reality she encountered in practice. She asked *'What occasions the distress (I and patients) experience?'* and diagnosed disempowerment.

Tessa has now taken a post in the School of Applied Social Science at the University of Brighton, a large component of which is nursing-related, and has, for the moment at least, staked a claim to a place in the field she had left. In *her* quest, and questioning, I see Tessa as part of the tradition I have tried to describe in this chapter. The tradition passes through Edinburgh. She, like Annie, displays what MacIntyre called '. . . an additional virtue . . . the virtue of having an adequate sense of the traditions to which one belongs or which confront one . . . [An] adequate sense of tradition manifests itself in a grasp of those future possibilities which the past has made available to the present. Living traditions, just because they continue a not-yet-completed narrative, confront a future whose determinate and determinable character, so far as it possesses any, derives from the past' (AV 223; MacIntyre 1985).

The task those in the tradition now face as nurses, teachers, students and scholars is to sustain 'an adequate sense of tradition' so as to 'grasp . . . future possibilities' of relationship with persons suffering from mental distress, based on affinity with them and a live hermeneutic of ethics and knowledge. One thing is constant: in our work we hold each other accountable for realising the goods of this tradition.

References

Allan, S. (1990) *Fear Not to Sow: A Life of Elsie Stephenson*. Newmill, Penzance, Cornwall: Jamieson Library.

Altschul, A. (1960:2001a) Report on the one-to-one relationship with Mrs. X, Boston. In: Altschul, A. (2001) *A Festschrift for Annie Altschul*, Paper 5, pp. 61–4. Edinburgh: Department of Nursing Studies, University of Edinburgh, and Royal College of Nursing.

Altschul, A. (1960:2001b) Feedback to supervisor, June Mellow, on one-to-one relationship with Mrs X. In: Altschul, A. (2001) *A Festschrift for Annie Altschul*, Paper 6, pp. 65–7. Edinburgh: Department of Nursing Studies, University of Edinburgh, and Royal College of Nursing.

Altschul, A. (1961:2001a) Report on a tour of the United States of America, Canada and Australia to study psychiatric nursing. May 1960–April 1961. Report to the Commonwealth Fund. In: Altschul, A. (2001) *A Festschrift for Annie Altschul*, Paper 2, pp. 2–36. Edinburgh: Department of Nursing Studies, University of Edinburgh, and Royal College of Nursing.

Altschul, A. (1961:2001b) Evaluation of one term at Boston University School of Nursing. In: Altschul, A. (2001) *A Festschrift for Annie Altschul*, Paper 4, pp. 50–60. Edinburgh: Department of Nursing Studies, University of Edinburgh, and Royal College of Nursing.

Altschul, A. (1964) *Aids to Psychiatric Nursing*, 2nd edn., p. 3. London: Baillière, Tindall and Cox.

Altschul, A. (1967) *Measurement of patient–nurse interaction in relation to in-patient psychiatric treatment*. Unpublished MSc (Social Science) dissertation, University of Edinburgh.

Altschul, A.T. (1972) *Patient–Nurse Interaction: A Study of Interaction Patterns in Acute Psychiatric Wards*. Edinburgh: Churchill Livingstone.

Altschul, A.T. (1973) A multidisciplinary approach to psychiatric nursing. *Nursing Times*, 69: 508–511.

Altschul, A. (1983) *The Effectiveness of the Community Psychiatric Services Provided by Dingleton Hospital for Psychogeriatric Patients in the Borders*. Edinburgh: Scottish Office Home and Health Department.

Altschul, A. (1997) A personal view of psychiatric nursing. In: *The Mental Health Nurse: Views of Practice and Education* (ed. S. Tilley), pp. 1–14. Oxford: Blackwell Science.

Altschul, A. (1999) Editorial. *Journal of Psychiatric and Mental Health Nursing*, 6 (4): 261–3.

Berger, P.L. & Luckmann, T. (1971) *The Social Construction of Reality: A Treatise in the Sociology of Knowledge*. Harmondsworth: Penguin.

Costello, J.E. (2002) *John Macmurray: A Biography*. Edinburgh: Floris.

Frank, A.W. (2000) The standpoint of storyteller. *Qualitative Health Research*, 10 (3): 354–65.

Greenblatt, M., York, R.H. & Brown, E.L., in collaboration with Hyde, R.W. (1955) *From Custodial to Therapeutic Patient Care in Mental Hospitals: Explorations in Social Treatment*. New York: Russell Sage Foundation.

John, A.L. (1960) *A study of the psychiatric nurse and his/her role in the care of the mentally ill*. Unpublished PhD dissertation, University of Edinburgh.

John, A.A. (1961) *A Study of the Psychiatric Nurse*. Edinburgh: E. & S. Livingstone.

MacDonald, D.J. & Altschul, A. (1972) *Study of the Multi-disciplinary Approach to Psychiatric Treatment Provided by Dingleton Hospital in the Border Counties*. Melrose: Board of Management of Dingleton Hospital.

MacIntyre, A. (1985) *After Virtue: a Study in Moral Theory*. London: Duckworth.

MacIntyre, A.F. (1989) Epistemological crises, dramatic narrative and the philosophy of science. In: *Anti-Theory in Ethics and Moral Conservatism* (eds S.A. Clark & E. Simpson), pp. 241–61. Albany: SUNY Press.

Macmurray, J. (1957) *The Self as Agent*. London: Faber and Faber.

Macmurray, J. (1964) Nurses in an expanded Health Service. *Nursing Mirror*, 8, 8 May: 113–15; 15 May: 135–7.

Mellow, J. (1964) *Evolution of nursing therapy and its implications for education*. Unpublished EdD dissertation, Boston University School of Education.

Parkes, T. (1997) Reflections from the outside in: my journey into, through and beyond psychiatric nursing. In: *The Mental Health Nurse: Views of Practice and Education* (ed. S. Tilley), pp. 58–72. Oxford: Blackwell.

Parkes, T. (2002) *Feathers and thorns: the politics of participation in mental health services*. Unpublished PhD dissertation, University of Kent at Canterbury.

Pollock, L. (1988) *Community psychiatric nursing explained: an analysis of the views of patients, carers and nurses*. Unpublished PhD dissertation, University of Edinburgh.

Pollock, L.C. (1989) *Community Psychiatric Nursing: Myth and Reality*. Harrow: Scutari.

Ryan, D. (1985) The professional and the personal: are they incompatible? In: *Accountable Autonomy: Perspectives in Professional Education* (ed. S. Goodlad), pp. 56–75. SRHE Annual Conference 1984. Guildford: Society for Research into Higher Education.

Schrock, R. (1981) *An argument concerning the meaning and relevance of philosophical enquiries in nursing*. Unpublished PhD dissertation, University of Edinburgh.

Sladden, S. (1977) *Psychiatric community nursing: a study of a working situation*. Unpublished PhD dissertation, University of Edinburgh.

Sladden S. (1979) *Psychiatric Nursing in the Community: A Study of a Working Situation*. Edinburgh: Churchill Livingstone.

Smith, H. (1982) *Beyond the Post-Modern Mind*. New York: Crossroad.

Tilley, S. (1990) *Negotiating realities: making sense of interaction between patients diagnosed as neurotic and nurses in two psychiatric admission wards*. Unpublished PhD dissertation, University of Edinburgh.

Tilley, S. (1995) *Negotiating Realities: Making Sense of Interaction Between Patients Diagnosed as Neurotic And Nurses*. Aldershot: Avebury.

Tilley, S. (1997) The mental health nurse as rhetorician. In: *The Mental Health Nurse: Views of Practice and Education* (ed. S. Tilley), pp. 152–171. Oxford: Blackwell Science.

Tilley, S. (1998) *Sustaining varieties of practice*. Invited keynote paper at English National Board National Mental Health Nursing Conference, Cambridge, England, 29–30 June 1998.

Tilley, S. (1999a) Discourses on empowerment. *Journal of Psychiatric and Mental Health Nursing*, 6 (1): 53–60.

Tilley, S. (1999b) Altschul's legacy in mediating British and American psychiatric nursing discourses: common sense and the 'absence' of the accountable practitioner. *Journal of Psychiatric and Mental Health Nursing*, 6 (4): 283–95.

Tilley, S. (2002) Annie Altschul – an appreciation. *Journal of Psychiatric and Mental Health Nursing*, 9 (2): 127–129.

Tilley, S. & Pollock, L. (2001) *Prudent Empowerment, Sustaining Relationships: Themes in Community Psychiatric Nurses' Work with People with Enduring Mental Disorders*. Edinburgh: Department of Nursing Studies, University of Edinburgh.

Weir, R.I. (1996) *A Leap in the Dark*. Newmill: Jamieson Library.

Chapter 4

Nursing Mental Health at the Tavistock

Peter Griffiths and Vicky Franks

Introduction

In this chapter we attempt to show how psychiatric and mental health nursing is constituted at the Tavistock Clinic. We begin by outlining the historical context of the Tavistock Clinic, its work and the recent development of the discipline of nursing within this academic and clinical institution. We draw attention to an older established field of psychodynamic and social systemic nursing knowledge, from which this 'new discipline' has emerged; and attempt to identify, albeit briefly, its distinguishing theoretical and practice positions, referencing relevant texts where appropriate. We then position this field of knowledge and practice within the wider field of mental health nursing, general nursing and developments more generally within the health care system. We have attempted to consider reflexively the influence of the institutions in which we work (the Tavistock Clinic and Middlesex University) on our role as knowledge producers. We identify some of the conflicting aspects of these roles and the associated contested fields of knowledge within both institutions. Lastly, we explore how we believe our particular field of experiential knowledge has enabled us to better navigate our roles, and offer a model to the nurse practitioners alongside whom we work, teach and learn.

Historical context

The evolution of nursing at the Tavistock Clinic

The Tavistock Clinic was founded in 1920 for the out-patient treatment of nervous disorders. The Children's Department of the clinic provided the model for child guidance clinics. Over the years it has developed to provide psychotherapeutic treatment for individuals, children, adolescents, families and groups. The work of the clinic is based on the application of psychoanalytic and systemic ideas to understanding human growth, psychological development and discontinuities and difficulties in these processes and in group and social processes both within the family and within wider society. In 1948 it became part of the

National Health Service. In 1995 it joined with the Portman Clinic (which provides treatment and training in forensic psychotherapy) to form the Tavistock and Portman NHS Trust.

The Tavistock Clinic's contribution to the study of institutions and organisational processes has gained international reputation through the work of the Tavistock Institute (previously a department of the Clinic) (Trist & Murray 1990), and more recently through the applied work of the Clinic, including institutional consultations (Obholzer & Roberts 1994).

The clinic is essentially divided into three major departments: the Adult, Adolescent, and Child and Family Departments. Within each of these there exist the disciplines of Psychiatry, Psychoanalytic Psychotherapy (adult, child and adolescent), Systemic Psychotherapy, Educational and Clinical Psychology, Social Work and Nursing. An integration of approaches from these disciplines underlies the range of work undertaken, developed and researched.

The Tavistock Clinic is a national and international training institution, where training and research are firmly based in the clinical practice. Applied psychotherapeutic training is based upon in-depth reflection and application of theory to students' own professional practice. Students use detailed observations from their own work settings, for discussion and exploration within practice discussion seminars during training. The clinic offers professional training to psychiatrists, educational psychologists, child psychotherapists, adult psychotherapists and systemic psychotherapists. Some of the courses are formal trainings in psychodynamic psychotherapy or systemic psychotherapy for the aforementioned disciplines. However, the majority are applications of these ideas, for use by professionals working within their core professions, or offered to allied professional workers from health, education, social services, the church, the probation service and the voluntary and charitable sector. Universities, which work in collaboration with the clinic, now validate academically most of the applied educational programmes and specific professional training courses.

Nursing as a distinct discipline within the Tavistock Clinic began in 1995 with the appointment of the first Senior Lecturer in Nursing. Shortly after this an MSc programme in applied psychodynamic practice was established, in collaboration with the Cassel Hospital and the Nursing School at Middlesex University. This was specifically created for nurses, social workers and other care professionals to provide a postgraduate education and training in the application of psychodynamic and social systemic ideas to practice in the settings from which students came. Over the last five years, more nurses have been appointed to Senior Lecturer posts, in different departments.

In June 2001 the Centre for Mental Health in Nursing (CMHN) was launched. The aim of the CHMN is to develop new models of psychotherapeutic mental health nursing for a range of different nurses working across the age range, from birth to old age, by applying psychodynamic and systemic thinking to the task (Franks & Griffiths 2001). These models are intended for established mental health nurses working in acute and community settings, and for nurses whose work already involves significant mental health work, but who have had very little preparation for this work in pre- or post-basic training. The latter might include midwives, health visitors, school nurses, practice nurses, district nurses, paediatric nurses or Accident and Emergency nurses (English National Board 2000a; UKCC 2000). The training will enable practitioners to develop the appropriate psycho-therapeutic skills and capabilities they need for this work (DoH 1999a, b). The models will involve moving beyond medication and remedial action, to working towards significant change and development in clients; aiming to promote mental health and prevent mental illness as well as care for and treat existing mental ill health.

Through its links with Middlesex University, the CMHN both runs and plans to develop further courses at Introductory, Advanced Diploma, Masters and Doctorate levels. It also aims to research practice and the effectiveness of training in developing practice, and establish a body of knowledge related to the subject. Ultimately there are plans to expand education and training into other parts of the country, as part of the Tavistock's National Training remit. New areas of work in nursing will link into existing training, clinical, consultation and research work undertaken within the Tavistock Clinic.

Further aims of the centre include:

- training supervisors and managers
- providing consultancy for nurses
- research, particularly into practice developments
- disseminating the outcomes of research and thinking via publications and papers
- influencing the working conditions and organisational cultures of nurses engaged in mental health work, to ensure that they are adequately supported to carry out this vital work
- local and national policy development.

The title, Centre for Mental Health in Nursing, was chosen to emphasise the contribution it is felt that the Tavistock paradigm of nursing can make to psychiatric mental health nursing (PMHN) and more generally to the mental health of nursing and nurses across all fields of nursing.

Nurses have undertaken training at the Tavistock Clinic for many years, attending a range of courses. However, this formerly 'invisible college' is now growing and has been made much more explicit within the institution, both by the employment of Nursing Lecturers in the early 1990s and by the validation of seven Tavistock courses as English National Board of Nursing (ENB) post-registration training courses.

Until very recently, views and beliefs about nurses, the profession of nursing, and the applicability and utility of psychodynamic and systemic ideas to nursing have been promulgated by course tutors from other disciplines within the Clinic. Tavistock course tutors have gained a knowledge of nursing through teaching nurses and through reviewing and exploring their professional experience with them (and of course through their own professional training and professional experience outside the clinic). The Tavistock has researched nurses and nursing experience, perhaps most notably in the work of Isabel Menzies-Lyth (Menzies 1970) but equally in work by others (Woodhouse & Pengelly 1991; Miller 1993; Obholzer & Roberts 1994; Foster & Roberts 1998).

Yet nursing, as a discipline, has only recently been accepted into the Tavistock Clinic as a co-discipline, 75 years after the Clinic was established. This has no doubt been driven by political and economic motivations, as well as by the sincerely held belief of some senior Tavistock staff (many of whom have worked with nurses in other settings, such as the Cassel Hospital) that nurses could both gain from and enrich the multi-disciplinary milieu at the clinic.

Anna Dartington (formerly a Cassel nurse who retrained as a social worker and was employed as such by the Tavistock) was influential in paving the way for the emergence of nursing as a discipline at the clinic. This was brought about through her continued interest in nursing, provision of a course for nurses at the Tavistock in the 1980s, and work with Julia Fabricius (1995) amongst others. In an analysis of the experience of nursing and of its effects upon others, she suggests:

> The intense emotions aroused [in nursing] are felt to threaten not only efficiency, but also the fabric of the institution itself . . . it seems to be the fate of those who work on the staff/client boundary to carry and attempt to contain this anxiety so that the rest of the organisation can experience an emotion-free zone in which to operate. In order to maintain this, these frontline workers must be silenced, anaesthetised, infantilized or otherwise rendered powerless. (Dartington 1994: 109)

Whilst the Tavistock is not in any way an emotion-free zone, one can perhaps hypothesise from comments about nurses and nursing made by colleagues from other disciplines that, for a considerable time, nursing was kept at arm's length for this reason. The Tavistock paradigm of nursing, as developed by nurses, is in many ways a new and emergent development at the Clinic. Whilst the Tavistock Clinic is imbued with a rich discourse in psychodynamic and social systemic ideas, it is perhaps accurate to suggest that the application of these ideas to nursing has until recently found its fullest expression outside the Clinic, in other institutions. As we will outline, Tavistock nursing draws its authority from a rich cultural history of psychodynamic and social-systemically informed nursing practice, developed over the years in diverse settings.

Psychodynamic nursing – models of practice

An adequate narrative history of this discourse within nursing has been neither fully described nor researched, though various nursing authors have made attempts at beginning this (Winship 1995a; Wright 1996; Griffiths & Leach 1998). Wright (1996) emphasises that culture does not reside solely in the present, nor is it a property of any one individual. Indeed it might be said that this cultural discourse within nursing has many surfaces of emergence (Foucault 1965, 1973,

1987), nationally and internationally. These points of emergence on occasions connect and yet sometimes seem to parallel each other but remain unrelated.

Perhaps the most well-known application of psychoanalytic thinking to nursing practice is contained within Hildegard Peplau's work on nursing, grounded in her work at Chestnut Lodge (an inpatient psychotherapy unit in the USA). Barker (1995) suggests that she was influenced by Erica Fromm and Harry Stack Sullivan, though she never worked directly with the latter. There were other centres within the USA such as Austin Riggs in Texas and the Menninger Clinic in Minnesota, where nursing informed by a psychodynamic perspective was developed. However, it was Peplau who most explicitly developed and advocated a psychoanalytic approach to nurses' work with psychiatric patients, believing that the interactive phenomena that occurred during nurse–patient relationships have a qualitative impact on outcomes for patients (Peplau 1952).

She reiterated this approach in the mid-1990s when she suggested that psychiatric nurses should include 50-minute, scheduled talking 'sessions' with their patients three days a week (Peplau 1994: 5). Yet it is important to note that this approach involves nurses adopting an additional profession, psychoanalytic psychotherapy, rather than applying psychodynamic theory in their everyday nursing practices. However, Winship rightly points out that Peplau maintained:

> It is the nurse herself who is the agent of change for a patient rather than the mechanism or the type of therapy. (Winship 1995a: 295)

Peplau's model has been influential in mental health nursing theory, but perhaps less so in practice, especially in the UK. It is an eclectic model, inductively derived and influenced by theory and theorists, from disciplines other than nursing. Nurses are seen as having an educative, therapeutic and maturing (nurturing) role: as counselling educators who deal with and resolve complex interpersonal issues (such as transference and counter-transference) in the process. In the model, a heavy emphasis is placed on psychodynamics and interpersonal dynamics (in the nurse-patient dyad). Peplau perhaps undervalued and underdeveloped the psychosocial and socio-cultural dimensions of the patient's human condition, the nurse's work and the setting. She acknowledges this herself in the preface to the third edition *Interpersonal Relations in Nursing* (Peplau 1988).

These ideas took root extensively in the USA. Under the influence of Peplau and others, Shirley Smoyak and Suzanne Lego (Lego 1992, 1998) – both pupils and then colleagues of Peplau – influenced the content of postgraduate mental health nurse training philosophically (Forchuk & Reynolds 1998). Yet Barker suggests that at the level of implementation in practice, Peplau had only limited impact in the USA and that her ideas have remained relatively marginally known in the UK (Barker 1998) and have often been criticised unfairly (cf. Gournay 1996). Whilst we would not wish to pursue this argument here, we are left with the impression that an explicit psychoanalytically-informed model of mental health nursing – as distinct from one that amounts to nurses becoming psychotherapists – was not attempted.

Psychodynamic nursing – therapeutic communities

In the UK, the influence of psychoanalytic ideas on the nursing profession as a whole has been comparatively weak. Influence has been greatest within the therapeutic communities in which nurses have worked. Whilst many of these have come and gone (see Pines 1979 for an exploration of this), therapeutic communities employing nurses, such as the Cassel and Henderson Hospitals have endured.

Wright (1996) identifies the subtle interactions between different nurses who worked and trained within these institutions, influenced by psychoanalysts within them, often by their own analysis, but most significantly by the cultures in which they worked, trained and developed their ideas. These were trainings based very much on an apprenticeship-type model of learning: learning from and through nursing experience. This type of learning was facilitated by the provision of formal, regular spaces for reflection on professional experience, throughout the working day, whilst the experience remained emotionally resonant and open to enquiry (Barnes 1968). Among nurses thus influenced were Doreen Waddell, who worked with Main and others at the Cassel; Elisabeth Barnes, who worked first at the Cassel, then at the Henderson, King's Fund and *Nursing Times*; and Eileen Skellern, who worked first at the Cassel (and shared a flat with Isabel Menzies-Lyth), then at the Henderson, and finally at the Maudsley Hospital, where she was Matron.

Annie Altschul developed her passion for psychiatric nursing at Mill Hill Military Psychiatric Hospital, where she began her psychiatric training in 1943. Dr Maxwell Jones was the Medical Superintendent and after World War II he moved to the Belmont Hospital (later renamed the Henderson Hospital) to further develop his ideas. Altschul returned to the Maudsley Hospital after the war but was profoundly affected by this formative experience, which Nolan suggests influenced her and her contemporaries for the rest of their professional lives (Nolan 1993: 101).

Wright (1996) draws attention to the significant intergenerational influence of these practitioners on himself and on other nurses. Regrettably little has been published about the development of the ideas which have informed nursing at the Henderson Hospital. The Cassel Hospital has been more productive. This has perhaps been influenced by the establishment of the course in psychosocial nursing at the Cassel and the associated academic rigour with which nurses were expected to write about their work and practice.

Following on from the early therapeutic community experiments at Northfield Military Hospital during World War II (Ahrenfeldt 1958; Main 1983; Bridger 1985; Harrison 1999), Tom Main, with Waddell, pioneered an action-based assessment and treatment model at the Cassel Hospital. This model integrated a practical use of psychoanalysis and social systems theory within a residential setting. This psychosocial treatment model involved the development of a language for understanding and practice, and the use of actions and activity, as well as words and phantasies (and their social representations).

Through ongoing development and the application of therapeutic community principles (Main 1946; Barnes 1968), the Cassel developed what it called a 'culture of enquiry' (Main 1983). This was a culture that set out actively to use the totality of the daily domestic and recreational aspects of living in the service of the therapeutic work, so that the reasons for difficulties, anxieties, failures and successes in these ordinary but fundamentally important aspects of patients' everyday life could be explored and discussed (Kennedy 1997). This discourse of thinking and practice evolved and developed out of the often challenging and difficult work the hospital undertook with patients including children, adolescents, adults and families presenting with severe emotional difficulties. An ongoing exploration of the interpersonal dynamics of this experience has led to the development of nursing practices that enable nurses to engage in this emotionally difficult work (Main 1957; Waddell, D. 1968; Chapman 1987, 1988a, b).

A formal nurse training began at the Cassel in 1951, for nurses interested in nursing patients with neurotic disturbances (Barnes 1968). This evolved into two kinds of training: short intensive courses for nurses of various grades and from different fields of practice, and an 18-month course for nurses of ward sister status. The latter course evolved over a period of almost 50 years into an internally certificated course in Psychological and Family-Centred Nursing. In 1994, the 18-month course was redeveloped as an accredited two-year full-time Diploma in Psychosocial Nursing, and validated with Manchester University. The original motivation for the development of these courses was to feed back into the nursing profession nursing experience gained at the Cassel Hospital. In particular, the aim was to develop an understanding of patients as individuals, and an understanding of their interactions and roles within their families, within groups and as members of a larger hospital community. A related aim was the development of identification and understanding of the psychological and emotional difficulties such patients had in relating to and functioning within such relationships and settings, and of the nursing practices that might therapeutically be brought to bear on these. Nurses undertaking these courses came from both general and psychiatric nursing backgrounds.

Mental health and ill health were not considered within the nosology of psychiatric classification, but instead within a framework that considered the problematic quality of personal and interpersonal relationships the individual or family manifest in their relationships with and to others. Mental health and ill health were perceived as relational to one's sense of self and in relation to one's relationships with and to others. To quote Rickman (cited by Winnicott):

> Mental illness consists in not being able to find anyone who can understand you. In other words there is a contribution from society into the meaning of the word ill. (Winnicott 1965: 218)

Mental disorder was believed to be most productively seen, in most instances, in psychological terms – as a product of specific beliefs, desires, emotions, intentional states and dysfunctional coping mechanisms both conscious and unconscious. It was felt that if one did not understand mental ill health in this way, it would be impossible to understand the all-too-evident psychosocial pathways to mental disorder: poverty, unemployment, incest, homelessness, violence, the heartlessness of abusive parenting and the innumerable methods people can find to inflict misery on one another. All of these experiences can influence people's relational expectations of others, the trust they may be capable or incapable of feeling, their expectations of care or its absence, within the family and later from professional carers.

A good deal has been written about psychosocial nursing over the years, and some of this has been published (Waddell, D. 1955; Barnes 1968; Haque 1973; Macklin 1979; De Lambert 1982; Chapman 1984, 1988a, b; Kennedy *et al.* 1987; Denford and Griffiths 1993; Flynn 1993; McCaffrey 1994, 1998; Robinson 1994; Simpson 1994; Irwin 1995; Griffiths and Pringle 1997; Pringle 1998, 1999; Pringle and Chiesa 2001). In 1998 Barnes *et al.* made the first attempt to develop an explicit model of psychosocial nursing practice, elaborating Cassel nurses' application of these ideas and developments within other health, social care and educational settings.

Psychodynamic nursing – the dissemination of ideas

Over the years various groups of interested nurses, some influenced by nurses who worked in the aforementioned institutions, established groups to further the utilisation of psychoanalytic ideas within nursing practice. Several hospitals (and now universities) have developed and run the ENB 660 one-year course in the application of psychodynamic ideas to nursing. The Nurses' Association for Psychodynamic Psychotherapy (NAPP) was established in the 1980s to secure the right of nurses to practise psychotherapy within the NHS. The Royal College of Nursing had for a while a Psychodynamic Education Group (PEG) and ran a Certificated Therapeutic Communities Course in association with the Association of Therapeutic Communities (the PEG, and the course, no longer exist).

In 1990, the newly established Association for Psychoanalytic Psychotherapy Therapy in the NHS (APP) ran a conference entitled 'Ethics and Emotions in Nursing' and, through the conference was poorly attended, a number of fascinating papers were published identifying the usefulness and relevance of psychoanalytic thinking to the understanding and application of nursing practice (Conran 1991; Fabricius 1991a; Goldie 1991; Wright 1991). Wright, influenced by Eileen Skellern at the Maudsley during his Registered Mental Nurse (RMN) training, went on to train at the Cassel. He later influenced this discourse significantly through a number of publications directed at pre- and post-registration nurses (Wright 1989; Wright & Giddy 1993).

More recently the APP has established a nursing subdivision and this runs regular seminars that explore the application of psychoanalytic and psychodynamic ideas to nursing practice, as well as an annual conference. Within these seminars, there have been many presentations where these ideas have been developed in conventional mental health and general nurse settings, yet rarely have these been written up for publication. More generally there have been very few applications of these ideas to nursing practice published by nurses. There are a few notable exceptions: Hughes and Halek (1991); Winship (1995a, b, 1998); Winship *et al.* (1995); Teising (2000); Wells *et al.* (2000). Perhaps Winship's conclusion still holds true, when in his review of the relationship between nursing and psychoanalysis he suggests:

> The relationship between psychoanalysis and nursing is still far from well defined, and for the most part, psychoanalytic ideas are perceived with some antipathy by the majority of nurses. (Winship 1995a: 289)

Whilst some nurses do regard these ideas with some antipathy (Gournay 1995b), it might be more accurate to conclude that many nurses have either never come across them in their studies or been only partially introduced to them, in a very limited way. As we have already indicated, there is not a large, coherent and integrated body of written work concerning the application of these ideas to nursing. Behavioural and cognitive approaches within PMHNing have been more thoroughly developed and researched.

Many aspects of psychodynamic nursing were introduced into the General Nursing Council (GNC) 1982 Syllabus of Training for Mental Health Nurses Guidelines, although its overarching theoretical paradigm was derived from humanistic psychology (General Nursing Council for England and Wales 1982). The syllabus emphasised the interpersonal nature of mental health nursing, the importance of the therapeutic relationship as an agent of therapeutic change and the possibilities of nurturing a therapeutic environment in mental health work. Nurse historians have seen this in part as the GNC's response to many of the criticisms made of mental health nursing care and practice in the plethora of inquiries and reports into maltreatment in psychiatric hospitals that characterised the 1960s and 1970s (Nolan 1993). However, the hasty introduction of this new syllabus two years before the Council was abolished, subsequent changes in nurse education, the movement of Schools of Nursing into Polytechnics/Colleges, Project 2000, and other developments resulted in incoherent and piecemeal introduction of these guidelines.

Psychodynamic and social systemic ideas and theories about human development and human 'being' are, in our experience, rarely explored or taught in pre-registration or post-basic nurse training. The capacity of these ideas to provide a rich understanding requires that those who teach them have a 'feel' for their application within clinical settings, of which there have been few. Nurses undertaking a nursing degree course may in their studies receive a nominal lecture on Freud or Jung. Yet this does not constitute an active exploration of the application of psychodynamic social systemic theory to nursing practice (Barnes *et al.* 1998; Wells *et al.* 2000). Nor does it adequately represent the rich psychodynamic discourse that has developed in critical theory and clinical research (Frosh 1991; Elliot 1996; Holloway & Jefferson 2000) since these original thinkers developed their seminal theories.

Of the six nurses who are now employed at the Centre for Mental Health in Nursing (CMHN), two have considerable experience of work and training at the Cassel. Another colleague undertook (with Julia Fabricius) significant work with general nurses (Fabricius 1991b, 1995), and another came under the influence of Beatrice Stevens at the Maudsley Hospital (Jackson & Cawley 1992; Jackson & Williams 1994). All of the Senior Nurse Lecturers at the CMHN have done or are undertaking significant postgraduate training at the Tavistock Clinic.

Our knowledge base therefore arises from a number of sources: seminal experiences within our own professional careers, post-registration training- and postgraduate training at the Tavistock Clinic. It is also informed significantly by the teaching we undertake with students, the learning we derive from participating in students' applications of these ideas to their own practice settings, and our own clinical nursing practice at the clinic.

The distinguishing features of psychodynamic knowledge in mental health nursing

What universally connects and distinguishes the nursing endeavours discussed above, and more recent developments (Byrt 1999), are the importance given to the intrapsychic and interpersonal experience in nursing work, the importance of nursing in a nurturing environment, and the therapeutic potential for change and transformation for nurses and their patients considered to reside within such an environment.

What distinguishes the Tavistock nursing paradigm is a discourse based in psychodynamic and systemic meta-paradigms, which creates a framework within which nursing experience is thought about, explored and possibly reconstituted. It is perhaps important to distinguish this approach from the development of a systems approach to nursing, which has been well developed in Canada and the USA (Freidmann 1998; Forchuk & Park Dorsay 1999; Wegner & Alexander 1999; Wright & Leahey 2000) and more recently in Edinburgh (Whyte 1997). Whilst the Tavistock nursing paradigm draws on these perspectives, it incorporates them within a psychodynamic understanding. These ideas have to some extent been elucidated elsewhere (Griffiths & Leach 1998), but their development at the Tavistock Clinic is emergent and therefore can be only partially and briefly elaborated here.

A psychodynamic and systemic view of mental health

Central to the Tavistock paradigm is an understanding of the importance of human emotional development; the interplay of this ongoing development between our conscious and unconscious awareness of ourselves, from the earliest age; and the effect this has on us throughout life, in all our relationships (Rayner 1986; Waddell, M. 1998).

Mental health and mental illness are not perceived in simple opposition to one another, but rather as two separate continua (Trent 1992) or axes (Downie 1990) i.e., existing alongside one another. Mental illness/ill health within this frame- work is viewed in terms of the 'continuous' explanatory model of psychoanalysis. This has a less dichotomous basis than psychiatry's discontinuous model which clearly separates those defined as mentally ill and those defined as mentally healthy (Siegler & Osmond 1976). Disorders of behaviour are believed to be largely an outward expression of inner emotional conflicts. Symptoms have mean- ing and seemingly irrational ('or mad') behaviour can sometimes be understood, if its past/present unconscious origins can be made partially explicit (Evans 1995; Evans & Franks 1997).

This view of mental health also encompasses an understanding of relatively stable yet socially destructive personality disorders. The structure of the person- ality is formed as a protective mechanism against mental fragmentation in the face of early stressors. The robust and enduring nature of the internal uncon- scious landscape is seen as extremely resistant to change and such patients will often damage helpful relationships rather than risk change (Bateman *et al.* 2000). Unconscious processes are used as a means of both relieving and communicating emotional distress. Because the processes are unconscious, the recipient (nurse or other carer) will not always recognise the phenomenon and will register discom- fort in the presence of certain patients. This may unwittingly elicit an unhelpful or counterproductive response from the nurse, as she responds unconsciously to this communication.

An individual's or family's difficulties are largely expressed in relationships with other people, even if the illness, for example schizophrenia, has a more obvious genetic or biological origin. The emerging/emergent disturbance will be to some extent a re-enactment (by an individual, couple, family, group or community) of past experiences and perhaps dysfunctional coping strategies that have grown out of this experience. Intrapsychic, interpersonal and beha- vioural change may be possible through a registering of re-enactment, a working through, understanding and reconstruction of thoughts, feelings and acts (James 1987: 82).

Psychodynamic features of mental health nursing

Nurses can feel overwhelmed in facing and experiencing the sheer level of pain, despair, distress and invariably anger that emotionally disturbed children and adults manifest. Even more distressing for the nurse can be his or her experience of the patient's destructive refusal to be helped; a characteristic response of dam- aged children and adults which confounds the nurse's desire to care. Many nurses who do not have appropriate skills and support switch off from the issues ad- dressed, as they feel ill equipped to take them on. They retreat to a professional persona which involves managing the 'case', keeping a professional distance or following rigid interpretations of their role and task. They pursue physical/

biological concerns, at the expense of psychological issues, which often manifest through and on the patient's body (Simpson 1998).

All patients have the right to be listened to and understood at as deep a level as possible. We believe that psychodynamic concepts have the capacity to facilitate this understanding. If a full understanding is to be achieved it is important to develop a collaborative understanding with the whole person, not merely a relationship with the presenting symptoms, difficulties or underlying pathology. The potential for change can be more fully realised if the nurse believes in the existence and value of a psychosocial dimension to care, rather than seeing the provision of care as a one-to-one curative act determined by the performance of a particular skill or intervention by the 'active nurse' upon the 'passive patient' (Main 1975). An individual's best hope for change or transformation in a psychosocial difficulty may instead be located in one or more domains – physical, psychological or social – and at an individual, interpersonal, group or community level of intervention. Careful, detailed observation over time develops a body of clinical evidence from which, and within which, meaning may be found (Hinshelwood 1987; Griffiths & Hinshelwood 1997).

Patients' lived experience and psychological difficulties can be understood through both what is conscious and what is brought to conscious awareness over time, through systematic engagement with the patient, as person, in her or his psychosocial context. Nurses can use a psychodynamic frame of reference alongside this, to explore with the patient how previous experiences and events may be impinging on their present relationships with others and themselves. This may entail a consideration of what might be being manifested/communicated unconsciously, by a registering of the patient's transference to the treatment setting, other patients, their relatives; and/or through the nurse's counter-transference to the patient (which may be experienced positively or negatively). This is a nursing use of transference and its corollary, countertransference (Salzberger-Wittenberg 1970; Schroder 1985; Copley & Forryan 1987; James 1987; Hughes & Halek 1991; Holmes & Perrin 1997; O'Kelly 1998).

Nurses provide in this way a relational container (in Bion's (1970) sense) for psychological disturbance to be registered and empathised with. They also act as a model for the patient, whose own capacity for tolerating frustration, mental pain and reflective thought may be seriously impaired (Jackson 1993). This notion of psychological containment can be used in the service of systemic awareness, rather than simply as rules of conduct, physical containment or defensive rituals (Menzies 1970; Tonnesman 1979; Roberts 1994).

The nurse's (and colleagues') feelings about the patient and the experiences of the patient in relation to the nurse, others and the environment, if registered and used, can deepen and enhance the patients' sense of identity, and their understanding of difficulties and of others' knowledge and experience of them (Chapman 1984; James 1987; Denford and Griffiths 1993; Evans and Franks 1997). Every-day structures such as cleaning, cooking, play groups, social and leisure activities, which many patients have difficulty in undertaking or engaging in socially, can provide opportunities for revelation, exploration and therapeutic intervention

(Winnicott 1971; Flynn 1993; McCaffrey 1994, 1998; Irwin 1995; Griffiths & Pringle 1997).

Nurses can hold on to hope and hopefulness if they can own and contain their own omnipotent phantasies of absolute cure (and its converse, feelings of total impotence or failure), and if they can recognise that the possibility for change resides more fully within the psychosocial matrix, not with them alone (Meinrath and Roberts 1982; Dartington 1994; Roberts 1994). The reality of personal and professional limits and the possibility of saying 'No' challenge both the omnipotence of the professional carer and the desire for absolute dependency found in the regressed part of the patient.

Nurses need to develop a strong internal sense of their role and responsibility, and reflexive valuing of their professional experience, if they are to maintain a therapeutic presence that will enable them to detect and work with disturbance in patients. This form of nursing is more than a goal (outcome-oriented). It is an emergent process over time, aimed at the provision of 'good enough' (Winnicott 1965) nurture and care (the matrix for possible transformation), rather than (omnipotently sought) cure of a symptom or disease (Fabricius 1999; Menzies-Lyth 1999).

The nursing environment, that has to be created, actively managed and sustained, needs to be reliable, stable, safe and psychologically robust enough to allow for experimentation with some success and survivable failure. The environment needs to provide a sufficiently permissive climate in which challenging behaviour and feelings can be expressed and equally (and in turn) challenged by collective and mutual enquiry. As much as thoughts need to be valued, so too do feelings. Strong feelings need to be expressed, recognised, explored and contained.

Vicissitudes within the multidisciplinary team inside and outside the hospital/ treatment setting may resonate with the patient's disturbance and *vice versa* (Stanton & Schwartz 1954; Main 1957). Stress and strain are often conventionally seen as wholly undesirable phenomena, to be managed or eradicated. Resistance to facing the anxieties of the work often finds expression at a team and institutional level in complex and problematic team dynamics (Griffiths & Hinshelwood 2001). This can be experienced as bewildering and frustrating for the individual nurse (English National Board 2000b) when the rhetoric of 'collaboration and team work' rings hollow. Within the form of nursing described here, there is a belief that the experience of these phenomena is meaningful, and that these phenomena can communicate important elements of the staff's and the patient's social reality (Gabbard 1992).

If spaces can be created in which these communications can be registered and understood (Dartington 1994), they can be contained (rather than controlled) and used to inform subsequent action (Hughes & Pengelly 1997; Streeck 1997; Hawkins & Shohet 2000). In this way the sources of the original stress can become known, humanised and situated within a relational social context (Newton 1995) and thereby experienced as less overwhelming and less persecutory. Nurses need to develop the ability to think with others when under pressure to act or react, and to resist the pressure (whether internally or externally driven) to merely act and not think; to tolerate the uncertainty of not knowing and of 'appearing not to know'. There is a need to develop the capacity for disciplined self-examination and a resourcefulness to use this capacity in the service of the patient, through normal human behaviour.

All of these issues involve re-examining existing personal and professional responses and reworking the workplace within: an internalised space within our minds, filled with cherished professional assumptions, ideas and beliefs gained over years of training and professional experience. Ideas that we may no longer rationally possess become beliefs which may come to possess us, to the detriment of professional practice. Reworking these beliefs involves mixed and conflicted feelings, as nurses need to re-evaluate what they thought they knew, perhaps mourn overvalued beliefs and risk new ways of professional being.

The role of psychodynamic nursing within the wider field of mental health nursing

We have described the field of knowledge, its location and some distinguishing features. One particular feature of this knowledge is the containing framework it affords for understanding the context of the work.

Two major societal shifts, which have occurred in recent years, have had a profound impact on the working context of mental health in nursing. The first is the changing boundaries of work resulting from successive government and professional policy initiatives. A combination of cost-reduction economic policy and the ideology of community care has led to many ill people with physical and mental ill health now living at home, with their relatives taking a major part in providing their care. The emphasis on care in the community and shorter hospital stays for many forms of treatment has had serious emotional consequences for nurses, patients and their families (Altschuler 1997; Altschuler & Dale 1997). In addition, Practice Nurses, District Nurses, School Nurses and Health Visitors are increasingly finding themselves dealing with mental health issues in their work with children, adolescents, adults and their families; work for which they have received little or no preparation (DOH 1999b; English National Board 2000a). This is partly because Community Psychiatric Nurses have refocused their attention in order to concentrate on those with severe and enduring mental illness (DoH 1994). At a time of increasing societal and political change within the National Health and Social Services, we believe it is crucial that the psychological experiences of the patient and the nurse are critically held in mind and valued.

The second shift has been the use and proliferation of information technology and the impact this has had in creating the boundaryless 'acoustic space' between working individuals (Lawrence 1999). This has resulted in a transition in the relationship between organisation and work; from the organisation as a container of the work, to one where the work becomes a container of the organisation (Lawrence 1999).

One aspect of both these developments has been the changing level of workers' attachment to their work (Miller 1999). The workplace is no longer perceived to be a safe container and the worker's relation to it can become more guarded, calculated and cynical. The fate that befalls the dependency needs of the worker is of critical importance in work that involves managing the dependency needs of others (Obholzer & Roberts 1994). This is the case in work that often involves uncertain, ambivalent and conflicted interpersonal relationships for patients, their relatives and nurses charged with providing their care. Research into the reasons why nurses leave the profession indicates a growing sense among nurses that organisations do not care for the workers (Meadows *et al.* 2000). Paradoxically, because of the shifts described above, the workplace is less able to meet the dependency needs of workers, at a time when it commands more of their time and emotional energy; perhaps particularly in mental health work (Miller 1999).

Miller (1999) proposes an alternative to the culture of dependency, with the aim of developing autonomous, choice-making individuals who can engage collaboratively with others. It is our contention that nurses need to develop this capacity. However, this requires an understanding of the context of the work and the nature of the contact with disturbed individuals, which we have suggested can exert a pull away from thoughtful collaborative work into defensive work which alienates and distances nurses from their practice, colleagues and patients.

Such understanding, an amalgam of open systems and psychoanalytic theories, is the foundation of the Tavistock paradigm of clinical supervision and organisational consultancy (Palmer 2000). This working paradigm is used internationally and has been described in use in the public and private sectors (French & Vince 1999).

The influence of the institutions in which we work on our role as knowledge producers

The illusions and 'fuzziness' (Miller 1999) of internal and external boundaries and the effect of working within and outside subsystems of work roles are familiar to all of us. Our experience of the institutions within which we work, our roles as knowledge producers and how our work is understood by colleagues, is itself a case study of the field of knowledge. We would like to describe this in relation to our development as role models for the autonomous collaborative practitioner.

One of the institutions in which we work is the Tavistock Clinic, a national organisation committed to the dissemination and influence of psychodynamic and systemic thinking in mental health. We work therapeutically with patients and this is an important component of our role because it provides a rich experiential base to our developing field of knowledge. However, most of the activities with which we are involved there and in our other employing institution, Middlesex University, are about extending the field of knowledge into a wider context. As living, working examples of the use of the field of knowledge we seek to promote, we attempt to practise and model the tasks necessary to be effective knowledge producers. We believe that all nurses who aspire to be autonomous collaborative practitioners need to master these tasks, which are to:

- work across institutional/agency boundaries
- form an attachment to the work content
- reflect on self in relation to others
- teach and learn in applying theory to practice
- work with competing and complementary paradigms.

Work across institutional / agency boundaries

We both work for two employing institutions. One, the University, has the primary task of higher education; the other, the Tavistock Clinic, has the primary tasks of mental health training and therapeutic service provision. In each institution we tend to be associated with the values and missions of the other. This can mean that some of the unwanted aspects of one institution get split off and projected into the other. We as boundary workers can get caught up in this projective process and can feel that we have to account for the perceived failings of one institution when we are present in the other.

Our field of knowledge has been helpful in providing us with an understanding of some of this process. Our roles as knowledge producers in the university tend to be configured around our professional standing as nurses and therapeutic practitioners. This clinical practice is highly valued in an institution that struggles to make clinical links. Our field of knowledge is at times considered esoteric, as indeed it can be. It is part of our task to present this field in as accessible and useful a format as possible.

Our role as knowledge producers in the Tavistock tends to be configured around our professional identity as nurses. As indicated above, the nursing discipline at the Tavistock is new, and at present there are few posts. Therefore we are valued primarily for our experience and contact with the wider context of nursing and secondarily for our roles as therapeutic practitioners. We do not have to make our working theoretical paradigm accessible, as everyone working there is familiar with it. However, what we do have to work at is raising an awareness of nurses and nursing and the application of our field to the practice of nursing, both among our disciplinary colleagues and among the students we teach.

We define our presence as nurses within the Tavistock Clinic by taking part in multi-professional fora related to research and clinical work in mental health. In these, we experience from other disciplines a combination of curiosity about our difference and a genuine desire to encompass the nursing perspective. This co-exists with a more covert wish to keep things as they were, within the professional hegemony of the disciplines at the Tavistock prior to nursing. Nursing is such a recent addition (since 1995) and this may be a symptom of the ambivalence and rivalry that exists among all professional groups in the professional pecking order (Hughes & Pengelly 1997).

We have been helped quite considerably in our task of working across these two boundaries by the establishment of two mechanisms. The first was the creation of a joint liaison group between the University and the Tavistock Clinic. The second has been the creation of the National Centre for Mental Health in Nursing, a collaboration between both institutions which has enabled all involved to create a third unifying institution in the mind, linking the (sometimes concordant, sometimes not) aspirations of both institutions (Franks & Griffiths 2001). By these means the tensions around splitting and projection are also held and worked with at a senior level.

Form an attachment to the work content

The institution in our minds is an amalgam of the two employing institutions, the Centre and our links to other interested groups. This 'virtual' institution enables us to broaden our field of knowledge and extend into acoustic space. The programmes of teaching we are involved with in both employing institutions enable us to have contact with a wide variety of students from all over the UK. The MSc in Psychodynamic Practice has resulted in an enlarged network of nurses who work in this way. There are national networks of psychodynamic nurses, one being the Nurses Section of the Association of Psychoanalytic Psychotherapy in the NHS. This small but expanding group of nurses seeks to apply the theory and principles of psychodynamic theory to nursing. They have a web site, meet regularly and hold national conferences.

There are several informal networks; for example, a group of like-minded nurse consultants have formed a psychodynamic interest group. It can be comforting to remain in this attachment to our virtual institution, but we are aware that our field of knowledge is quite under-represented in mental health nursing. We are also aware of some misapprehensions about the current practice and application of psychoanalytic theory (Frosh 1997). There will always be rivalries and splits in any professional domain. We are mindful that our role as applied psychoanalytic knowledge producers in this domain will expose us to both idealisation and denigration. The working practice and application of psychoanalytic theory is frequently attacked as non-scientific, costly and time consuming, accessible to only a limited group of people (Holmes & Lindley 1989; Fonagy 2000a). If we are to function effectively as knowledge producers, we have to equip ourselves (and our students) with robust and convincing arguments for the validity of our approach (Rustin 2001). This means that we have to interact with others and debate the relevance of the unconscious, the importance of detailed observation, the use of feelings as evidence and the effectiveness of our field in promoting better relationships in mental health care. We have to be abreast of policy initiatives and the relevance of our understanding to national and international debates in mental health (Evans & Franks 1997; Griffiths 2001).

Reflect on self in relation to others

The need to tolerate not knowing and to reflect on self and others is central to our paradigm. This has meant that we need constantly to examine our working relationships in both employing institutions and our effectiveness in fulfilling the primary task in both. This is a crucial capacity and is recognised in nursing curricula (UKCC 2001) and in most clinical supervision approaches as essential to professional development (Hawkins & Shohet 2000).

Our paradigm also considers that relationships are central to the nursing task, and this is acknowledged to be essential in all nursing curricula (UKCC 2001). The nurse's use of self in managing relationships with colleagues and patients has been a recurrent theme in mental health nursing (Michael 1994; Barnes *et al.* 1998; Cutcliffe & McKenna 2000a, b), although occasionally it appears as something innovative and newly discovered, even in the national press (Brindle 2001)! However, the nurse's 'use of self', whilst a much exalted phrase, especially in psychiatric nursing textbooks, is not an easy process to define or practise, particularly when individuals' professional defences developed against this process are compounded by social defences against the often-messy interpersonal nature of the work (Obholzer & Roberts 1994).

The value of clinical supervision using a psychodynamic approach is such that this process can be explored. Unhelpful defences can be observed, made more manifest and worked on; and their anti-therapeutic properties can be addressed (Hughes & Pengelly 1997). Most clinical supervision models in nursing explicitly or implicitly use psychodynamic concepts; for example, the transference relationship, and the parallel between the process of supervisee/supervisor relationship and the patient/professional relationship.

Teach and learn in applying theory to practice

Learning involves unlearning and the uncertainty associated with this. This is painful, and if it cannot be tolerated it is often avoided (Main 2001). There can be a yearning for simple answers, reliance on which can squash curiosity (Salzberger-Wittenberg *et al.* 1983). We are aware that in our teaching we have to present students with very complex and abstract ideas. We too have to continue to learn in our own field. Deep personal reflection and a capacity to tolerate confusion help us in struggles to achieve this. It has meant that we experience some of the mental pain connected with learning and yet try to set an example of maintaining curiosity in the face of chaos, and hope in the face of despair. Our capacity to be reflective and thoughtful, rather than to produce ready answers, provides a model that enables our students to internalise a capacity for thinking for use in their own practice. Developing students' receptiveness to another person's communication depends on the teacher modelling a psychological willingness and capacity to be in touch with the feelings and thoughts of students, colleagues and patients. Some students will wish to rid themselves of their problems and dump them onto another person. Sometimes this is the teacher, from whom they expect ready, anxiety-relieving answers.

These psychodynamic insights assist us in the difficult task of being knowledge producers, particularly on programmes that seek to facilitate emotional as well as intellectual understanding. Knowledge of the process of learning in nursing has been described psychodynamically in relation to small group experiential work (Fabricius 1991b, Franks *et al.* 1994). The effect on the teacher has also been described by Fabricius in relation to lecturer liaison in clinical areas (Fabricius 1995).

Whilst we are aware of the seductive pull of simpler theories of psychic change (Milton 2001), we are also aware of the excitement (both negative and positive) that our teaching provokes. When we teach on the mental health branch of Project 2000, we notice that some students can become very animated and interested. It is as if they have found something different but quite profound, or perhaps rediscovered an aspect of their initial motivation for nursing: the wish to use their sense of self and personal experience in their professional work.

We believe that the breadth and depth of our explanatory framework are its most compelling qualities. It affords an explanation for the origins of emotions, a model of personality structure and a model for therapeutic change. In terms of therapeutic practice, it provides a rationale for what is often deemed irrational, especially in mental health work; and is frequently the treatment of choice for otherwise-untreatable patients with long-standing personality disorders (Bateman *et al.* 2000).

Work with competing and complementary paradigms

There are two distinct movements in clinical nursing. On the one hand there are those who advocate the technological advance of nursing care, the expansion of the nurse's role to include nurse prescribing, taking blood, etc.; on the other hand there are those who advocate a more relational approach. This is mirrored in the PMHNing field (Cutcliffe & Campbell 2002). Tilley (1997) coined the term 'care wars' (p. 204) to characterise the wider debate within PMHNing, which seems to centre on the search for a 'canonical text' and an authorised model of PMHNing.

The debate concerns the identities and associated practices in relation to which mental health/psychiatric nurses should position themselves. It is being conducted largely within mental health nursing academe (Fursland 1998), at a theoretical level. The 'care wars' debate ranges from a post-modernist critique of contemporary practice which advocates a more social-constructionist approach to mental health nursing (Clarke 1996; Stevenson 1996), to a critique of contemporary practice and advocacy of a more biochemical, genetically-orientated and instrumental approach (Gournay 1997). In this latter approach, nurses are exhorted to develop their role and professional identity as agents of medical treatment, for example by participating in the diagnosis of positive and negative symptoms in schizophrenia. They should gain medication-prescribing privileges and teach patients and families about the medical constructions of mental illness (Gournay 1995a, b). Morrall (1998) has suggested that mental health nurses should abandon the unrealisable goal of independent professionalisation, align themselves again with psychiatry and accept an explicit social control function.

The alternative position advocates that nurses should acknowledge that the phenomena they deal with, as nurses, are human responses to various life problems. From this position the nurse's main task should be to address people as human beings first, and patients with problems second (Barker 1997; Barker *et al.* 1997).

It may be that psychiatry/mental health has reached something of a crossroads (Clare 1999), but we do not believe that these are necessarily mutually exclusive routes for mental health (Fonagy 2000b) or for PMHNs. However, those who focus primarily on the alternative position are our natural allies. These nurses may be predominantly socio-political, philosophical, systemic, person-centred or cognitive in their approach. We have the same broad aim, which is to maintain the centrality of the nurse/patient/client/family relationship and its therapeutic potential in exploring the lived experience of the person/family in care, and as a medium for growth and development. A growing body of research indicates that it is the interpersonal, human person-to-person contact that patients want from their nurses, when mental health concerns predominate (Beech & Norman 1995; Cutcliffe *et al.* 1997; Mental Health Foundation 2000).

Within the Tavistock Clinic there are two complementary paradigms: systems theory and psychoanalytic theory. Campbell (1998) claims that the practitioner's choice of one or the other depends on where one locates the self, personally and professionally. If we locate self within our own skin, we become interested in the metaphor of the internal world and intrapsychic conflicts. On the other hand, if we locate our sense of self 'out there', we become interested in relational constructions and metaphors about interaction, such as feedback and reflexivity and dialogue between self and other. This may be one way of explaining why people choose a particular field in mental health, and their allegiance to one explanation rather than another. Certainly it can lead to intense rivalry and an inability to listen to another's viewpoint (Campbell 1998).

Within the university there is much greater diversity and allegiance to many different mental health approaches. This is often a matter of use of different languages or eclectic use of a number of them, but it may also be about holding different philosophical positions regarding the nature of man and knowledge. Within the School of Health and Social Science, one of our colleagues has a joint appointment between the School and the Sainsbury Centre for Mental Health. We are still exploring and clarifying the similarities and differences between our theoretical approach and his (Sainsbury Centre for Mental Health 2000).

Conclusions

It is a particular feature of our approach that conflict should not be avoided but instead should be worked with, and indeed that conflict can lead to greater creativity (Lousada 1998). Yet we need to remain vigilant to the ever-present shadows of competition and rivalry that can dull curiosity, the possibilities of creative intercourse and the development of practice most suited to the mental health needs of patients and practitioners.

We have suggested that our field can be either idealised or denigrated. This may simply be based on misconceptions due to confusing psychoanalysis as a distinct clinical discipline, with psychoanalytic theory as a discourse that can be applied in other ways by other people in their distinctive professions (Fonagy 2000a, b, Bell 2001). We have to be aware of this. We find that as knowledge producers in the university we are frequently called upon to defend and legitimise programmes that are largely psychodynamic and social-systemic. Our experience at the Tavistock enables us to understand that this is common to most practitioners who seek to apply psychoanalytic theory. It is part of the territory we inhabit. As knowledge producers we have to make clear the aforementioned distinction, unpick misconceptions and challenge prejudicial views. We readily take up the challenge, but at times find it is necessary to resist the temptation to retreat into a bunker mentality.

We believe that our field has much to offer current mental health nursing practice. However, we have much to learn from other approaches, and there is a growing rapprochement between our paradigm and others (Holmes 2000; Milton 2001).

We have described how our work as knowledge producers has enabled us to apply our field to our own practice as autonomous collaborative practitioners. We feel that our experience may serve as a model for all nurses who work in the wider field of current mental health practice.

Acknowledgement

We would like to acknowledge the help and support of Dr Harry Wright in the preliminary preparation of this chapter.

References

Ahrenfeldt, R.H. (1958) *Psychiatry in the British Army in the Second World War*. London: Routledge and Kegan Paul.

Altschuler, J. (1997) Family relationships during serious illness. *Nursing Times*, 93 (7): 48–49.

Altschuler, J. & Dale, B. (1997) The impact of illness on the family. In: *Working with Chronic Illness* (ed. J. Altschuler), Chapter 3. Basingstoke: Macmillan Press.

Barker, P. (1995) *Psychiatric nursing and psychoanalytic influences – historical perspectives*. Paper presented at the Association for Psychoanalytic Psychotherapy (APP) in the NHS Inaugural Nursing Sub-Committee Conference, 28 October 1995, London.

Barker, P. (1997) Towards a meta-theory of psychiatric nursing. *Mental Health Practice*, 1 (4): 18–21.

Barker, P. (1998) The future of the Theory of Interpersonal Relations? A personal reflection on Peplau's legacy. *Journal of Psychiatric and Mental Health Nursing*, 5: 213–220.

Barker, P.J., Reynolds, W. & Stevenson, C. (1997) The human science and basis of psychiatric nursing: theory and practice. *Journal of Advanced Nursing*, 25: 660–667.

Barnes, E. (ed.) (1968) *Psychosocial Nursing: Studies from the Cassel Hospital*. London: Tavistock.

Barnes, E., Griffiths, P., Ord, J. & Wells, D. (eds) (1998) *Face to Face with Distress: The Professional Use of Self in Psychosocial Care*. Oxford: Butterworth Heinemann.

Bateman, A., Pedder, J. & Brown, D. (2000) *Introduction to Psychotherapy: An Outline of Psychodynamic Principles and Practice*, 3rd edn. London: Routledge.

Beech, P. & Norman, I.J. (1995) Patients' perceptions of the quality of psychiatric nursing care: findings from a small descriptive study. *Journal of Clinical Nursing*, 4: 117–123.

Bell, D. (2001) *Psychoanalysis: a body of knowledge of mind and human culture*. Paper given to the Tavistock Scientific Meeting, 12 November 2001.

Bion, W. (1970) *Attention and Interpretation*. London: Tavistock.

Bridger, H. (1985) Northfield revisited. In: *Bion and Group Psychotherapy* (ed. M. Pines). London: Routledge and Kegan Paul.

Brindle, D. (2001) Active Service. *The Guardian*, Society Section, 7 November 2001, pp. 119–20.

Byrt, R. (1999) Nursing: the importance of the psychosocial environment. In: *Therapeutic Communities: Past, Present and Future* (eds R. Haigh & P. Campling), Chapter 5. London: Jessica Kingsley.

Campbell, D. (1998) *Ideas which divide the Tavistock: what are they really about?* Tavistock Clinic Paper no. 184. Presented to the Tavistock Scientific Meeting, 12 January 1998.

Chapman, G.E. (1984) A therapeutic community, psychosocial nursing and the nursing process. *International Journal of Therapeutic Communities*, 5: 68–76.

Chapman, G.E. (1987) Social action theory and psychosocial nursing. In: *The Family as In-patient* (eds R. Kennedy, A. Heymans & L. Tischler), Chapter 20. London: Free Association Books.

Chapman, G.E. (1988a) Reporting therapeutic discourse in a therapeutic community. *Journal of Advanced Nursing Studies*, 13: 255–64.

Chapman, G.E. (1988b) Text, talk and discourse in a therapeutic community. *International Journal of Therapeutic Communities*, 9 (2): 75–87.

Clare, A. (1999) Psychiatry's future: psychological medicine or biological psychiatry? *Journal of Mental Health*, 8 (2): 109–111.

Clarke, L. (1996) The last post? Defending nursing against the modernist maze. *Journal of Psychiatric and Mental Health Nursing*, 3: 257–65.

Conran, M. (1991) Running on the spot or can nursing really change? Response to Julia Fabricius. *Psychoanalytic Psychotherapy*, 5 (2): 109–114.

Copley, B. & Forryan, B. (1987) *Therapeutic Work with Children and Young People*. Part 5. The Therapeutic Relationship: Containment, Mental Pain and Thought, Chapter 13, and Transference and Countertransference, Chapter 15. London: Cassell.

Cutcliffe, J. & Campbell, P. (2002) Opinion: taking on nurse prescribing powers could lead mental health nurses away from core concepts that underpin nursing. *Mental Health Practice*, 5 (5): 14–17.

Cutcliffe, J. & McKenna, H. (2000a) Generic nurses: the nemesis of psychiatric mental health nursing, part 1. *Mental Health Practice*, 3 (9): 10–14.

Cutcliffe, J. & McKenna, H. (2000b) Generic nurses: the nemesis of psychiatric mental health nursing, part 2. *Mental Health Practice*, 3 (10): 20–23.

Cutcliffe, J.R., Dikintis, J., Carberry, J., *et al.* (1997) Users' views of their continuing care psychiatric services. *International Journal of Psychiatric Nursing Research*, 3: 382–94.

Dartington, A. (1994) Where angels fear to tread. In: *The Unconscious at Work* (eds A. Obholzer & V. Roberts), Chapter 13. London: Routledge.

De Lambert, L. (1982) The role of a nurse in a psychotherapeutic institution. In: *Psychotherapie in der Klinik*. Berlin: Springer.

Denford, J. & Griffiths, P. (1993) 'Transferences to the institution' and their effect on inpatient treatment at the Cassel Hospital. *Therapeutic Communities*, 14 (4): 237–48.

DoH (1994) *Working in Partnership: A Collaborative Approach to Care: Report of the Mental Health Nursing Review Team*. London: HMSO.

DoH (1999a) *Making a Difference: Strengthening the Nursing, Midwifery and Health Visiting Contribution to Health and Health Care*. London: DoH.

DoH (1999b) *A National Service Framework for Mental Health* (in particular Standards One Mental Health Promotion and Two Primary Care and Access to Services). London: DoH.

Downie, R. (1990) Ready, steady, stop? *Social Work Today*, 12 July 1990.

Elliot, A. (1996) *Subject to Ourselves: Social Theory, Psychoanalysis and Postmodernity*. Oxford, Polity.

English National Board (2000a) *Draft Report: Results of a Survey Undertaken to Establish the Extent to Which Pre-registration Nursing Programmes Address Child and Adolescent Mental Health*. London: ENB.

English National Board Research Highlight 40 (2000b) *Team Working in Mental Health: Zones of Comfort and Action*. London: ENB.

Evans, M. (1995) *The use of knowledge in nursing and psychotherapy as a defence against unbearable experiences*. Paper presented at the Association for Psychoanalytic Psychotherapy (APP) in the NHS Inaugural Nursing Sub-Committee Conference, 28 October 1995, London.

Evans, M. & Franks, V. (1997) Psychodynamics as an aid to clear thinking about patients. *Nursing Times*, 93 (10): 50–52.

Fabricius, J. (1991a) Running on the spot or can nursing really change? *Psychoanalytic Psychotherapy*, 5 (2): 97–108.

Fabricius, J. (1991b) Learning to work with feelings – psychodynamic understanding and small group work with junior nurses. *Nurse Education Today*, 11: 134–42.

Fabricius, J. (1995) Psychoanalytic understanding and nursing: a supervisory workshop with nurse tutors. *Psychoanalytic Psychotherapy*, 9 (1): 17–29.

Fabricius, J. (1999) The crisis in nursing. *Psychoanalytic Psychotherapy*, 13 (3): 203–206.

Flynn, C. (1993) The patients' pantry: the nature of the nursing task. *Therapeutic Communities*, 14 (4): 227–36.

Fonagy, P. (2000a) The hope of a future. *The Psychologist*, 13 (12): 620–23.

Fonagy, P. (2000b) Mind over molecules. *Mental Health Care*, 41 (31): 83.

Forchuk, C. & Park Dorsay, J. (1999) Hildegard Peplau meets family systems nursing: innovation in theory based practice. In: *Readings in Family Nursing* (eds G.D. Wegner & R.J. Alexander), Chapter 37. Philadelphia: Lippincott.

Forchuk, C. & Reynolds, B. (1998) Guest editorial – interpersonal theory in nursing practice: the Peplau legacy. *Journal of Psychiatric and Mental Health Nursing*, 5: 165–6. (The whole edition of this journal is given over to reviewing Peplau's influence on PMHN and is a useful source of reference.)

Foster, A. & Roberts, V. (1998) *Managing Mental Health in the Community: Chaos and Containment*. London: Routledge.

Foucault, M. (1965) *Madness and Civilization: A History of Insanity in the Age of Reason.* London: Tavistock.

Foucault, M. (1973) *The Birth of the Clinic: An Archaeology of Medical Perception.* London: Tavistock.

Foucault, M. (1987) *Mental Illness and Psychology.* Berkeley: California Press.

Franks, V. & Griffiths, P. (2001) Teaching emotional nursing. *Practice Nursing*, 12 (9): 351–3.

Franks, V., Watts, M. & Fabricius, J. (1994) Interpersonal learning in groups: an investigation. *Journal of Advanced Nursing*, 20: 1162–9.

Freidmann, M.L. (1998) *Family Nursing, Theory and Practice*, 4th edn. East Norwalk, Connecticut: Appleton-Lange.

French, R. & Vince, R. (eds) (1999) *Group Relations, Management and Organisation.* Oxford: Oxford University Press.

Frosh, S. (1991) *Identity Crisis: Modernity, Psychoanalysis and the Self.* Basingstoke: Macmillan.

Frosh, S. (1997) *For and Against Psychoanalysis.* London: Routledge.

Fursland, E. (1998) People. *Nursing Times*, 94 (24): 40–41.

Gabbard, G.O. (1992) The therapeutic relationship in psychiatric hospital treatment. *Bulletin of the Menninger Clinic*, 56 (1): 4–19.

General Nursing Council for England and Wales (1982) *Training Syllabus. Register of Nurses, Mental Nursing.* London: General Nursing Council for England and Wales.

Goldie, L. (1991) Ethical dilemmas for nurses and their emotional implications. *Psychoanalytic Psychotherapy*, 5 (2): 125–138.

Gournay, K. (1995a) New facts on schizophrenia. *Nursing Times*, 91: 32–3.

Gournay, K. (1995b) What to do with nursing models. *Journal of Psychiatric and Mental Health Nursing*, 2 (5): 325–7.

Gournay, K. (1996) Schizophrenia: a review of the contemporary literature and implications for mental health nursing theory, practice and education. *Journal of Psychiatric and Mental Health Nursing*, 3: 7–12.

Gournay, K. (1997) Responses to: 'What to do with Nursing Models' – a reply from Gournay. *Journal of Psychiatric and Mental Health Nursing*, 4: 227–31.

Griffiths, P. (2001) Child and adolescent mental health: a cause for concern in primary care nursing. *Mental Health Practice*, 5 (1): 38–9.

Griffiths, P. & Hinshelwood, R.D. (1997) Actions speak louder than words. In: *Psychosocial Practice in a Residential Setting* (eds P. Griffiths & P. Pringle), Chapter 1. London: Karnac Books.

Griffiths, P. & Hinshelwood, R.D. (2001) Enquirying into a culture of enquiry. In: *Reflective Enquiry in Therapeutic Institutions* (eds P. Griffiths & P. Pringle), Chapter 2. Cassel Monograph 2. London: Karnac Books.

Griffiths, P. & Leach, G. (1998) Psychosocial nursing: a model learnt from experience. In: *Face to Face with Distress: The Professional Use of Self in Psychosocial Care* (eds P. Griffiths & P. Pringle), Chapter 1. Oxford: Butterworth Heinemann.

Griffiths, P. & Pringle, P. (eds) (1997) *Psychosocial Practice in a Residential Setting.* London: Karnac Books.

Haque, G. (1973) Psychosocial nursing in the community. *Nursing Times*, 13 January.

Harrison, T. (1999) *Bion, Rickman, Foulkes and the Northfield Experiments: Advancing on a Different Front.* London: Jessica Kingsley.

Hawkins, P. & Shohet, R. (2000) *Supervision in the Helping Professions.* Buckingham: Open University Press.

Hinshelwood, R.D. (1987) *What Happens in Groups: Psychoanalysis, the Individual and the Community*. London: Free Association Books.

Holloway, W. & Jefferson, T. (2000) *Doing Qualitative Research Differently: Free Association, Narrative and Interview Method*. London: Sage.

Holmes, G. & Perrin, A. (1997) Countertransference: what is it? What do we do with it? *Psychodynamic Counselling*, 3: 263–77, 3 August.

Holmes, J. (2000) Attachment theory and psychoanalysis: a rapproachment. *British Journal of Psychotherapy*, 17 (2): 157–72.

Holmes, J. & Lindley, R. (1989) *The Values of Psychotherapy*. London: Karnac Books.

Hughes, P.M. & Halek, C. (1991) Training nurses in psychotherapeutic skills. *Psychoanalytic Psychotherapy*, 5 (2): 115–23.

Hughes, L. & Pengelly, P. (1997) *Staff Supervision in a Turbulent Environment*. London: Jessica Kingsley.

Irwin, F. (1995) The therapeutic ingredients in baking a cake. *Therapeutic Communities*, 16 (4): 263–8.

Jackson, M. (1993) Psychoanalysis, psychiatry, psychodynamics; training for integration. *Psychoanalytic Psychotherapy*, 7 (1): 7–14.

Jackson, M. & Cawley, R. (1992) Psychodynamics and psychotherapy on an acute psychiatric ward. *British Journal of Psychiatry*, 160: 41–50.

Jackson, M. & Williams, P. (1994) *Unimaginable Storms: A Search for Meaning in Psychosis*. London: Karnac Books.

James, O. (1987) The role of the nurse/therapist relationship in the therapeutic community. In: *The Family as In-patient* (eds R. Kennedy, A. Heymann & L. Tischler), Chapter 4. London: Free Association Books.

Kennedy, R. (1997) Work with the work of the day: the use of everyday activities as agents for treatment, change and transformation. In: *Psychosocial Practice in a Residential Setting* (eds P. Griffiths & P. Pringle), Chapter 2. London: Karnac Books.

Kennedy, R., Heymans, A. & Tischler, L. (1987) *The Family as In-patient*. London: Free Association Books.

Lawrence, W.G. (1999) A Mind for Business. In: *Group Relations, Management and Organisation* (eds R. French & R. Vince). Oxford: Oxford University Press.

Lego, S. (1992) Biological psychiatry and psychiatric nursing in America. *Archives of Psychiatric Nursing*, 5: 147–50.

Lego, S. (1998) The application of Peplau's theory to group psychotherapy. *Journal of Psychiatric and Mental Health Nursing*, 5: 193–6.

Lousada, J. (1998) The threat to clinical social work and the attack on linking. *Proceedings of the International Social Work Conference*, Florence, 14–16 March 1998.

Macklin, D. (1979) Trouble stirring in the kitchen. *Nursing Times*, 24 May.

Main, T.F. (1946) The hospital as a therapeutic institution. *Bulletin of the Menninger Clinic*, 10 (3): 66–70. Also republished in Johns, J. (1989) *The Ailment and Other Psychoanalytic Essays*. London: Free Association Press, pp. 7–11.

Main, T.F. (1957) The ailment. *British Journal of Medical Psychology*, 30: 129–45. Also republished in Johns, J. (1989) pp. 12–35.

Main, T. (1975) Some dynamics of large groups. In: *The Large Group* (ed. L. Kreeger), pp. 57–86. London: Constable. Also republished in Johns, J. (1989) pp. 100–22.

Main, T.F. (1983) The concept of a therapeutic community – variations and vicissitudes. In: *The Evolution of Group Analysis* (ed. M. Pines). London: Routledge and Kegan. Also republished in Johns, J. (1989) pp. 123–44.

Main, T.F. (2001) Knowledge, learning and freedom from thought. In: *Reflective Enquiry in Therapeutic Institutions* (eds L. Day & P. Pringle), Chapter 1. Cassel Monograph 2. London: Karnac Books.

McCaffrey, G. (1994) An account of outreach nursing at the Cassel. *Therapeutic Communities*, 15 (3): 173–81.

McCaffrey, G. (1998) The use of leisure activities in a therapeutic community. *Journal of Psychiatric and Mental Health Nursing*, 5 (1): 53–58.

Meadows, S., Levenson, R. & Baeza, J. (2000) *The Last Straw: Explaining the NHS Nursing Shortage*. London: King's Fund.

Meinrath, M.R. & Roberts, J. (1982) On being a good enough staff member. *International Journal of Therapeutic Communities*, 3: 7–14.

Mental Health Foundation (2000) *Strategies for Living*. London: MHF.

Menzies, I.E.P. (1970) *The Functioning of Social Systems as a Defence Against Anxiety*. Tavistock Pamphlet no. 3. The Tavistock Institute of Human Relations. London: Headley Brothers.

Menzies-Lyth, I. (1999) Facing the crisis. *Psychoanalytic Psychotherapy*, 13 (3): 207–212.

Michael, S. (1994) Invisible skills. *Journal of Psychiatric and Mental Health Nursing*, 1: 56–57.

Miller, E. (1993) Innovation in a psychiatric hospital. In: *From Dependency to Autonomy – Studies in Organisations and Change* (ed. E. Miller), Chapter 12. London: Free Association Books.

Miller, E. (1999) Dependency, alienation or partnership? The changing relatedness of the individual to the enterprise. In: *Group Relations, Management and Organization* (eds R. French & R. Vince). Oxford: Oxford University Press.

Milton, J. (2001) Psychoanalysis and cognitive behaviour therapy – rival paradigms or common ground? *International Journal of Psychoanalysis*, 82: 431–47.

Morrall, P. (1998) Mental health nursing and social control. *Mental Health Practice*, 11 (8): 12–13.

Newton, T. (1995) *'Managing' Stress, Emotion and Power at Work*. London: Sage.

Nolan, P. (1993) *A History of Mental Health Nursing*. London: Chapman and Hall.

Obholzer, A. & Roberts, V. (eds) (1994) *The Unconscious at Work: Individual and Organisational Stress in the Human Services*. London: Routledge.

O'Kelly, G. (1998) Countertransference in the nurse–patient relationship: a review of the literature. *Journal of Advanced Nursing*, 28 (2): 391–7.

Palmer, B. (2000) The Tavistock paradigm as a discursive practice. *Organisational and Social Dynamics*, 1 (1): 8–20.

Peplau, H.E. (1952) *Interpersonal Relations in Nursing*. New York: Putnam.

Peplau, H.E. (1988) Preface. *Interpersonal Relations in Nursing*, 3rd edn. London: Macmillan Education.

Peplau, H.E. (1994) Psychiatric mental health nursing: challenge and change. *Journal of Psychiatric and Mental Health Nursing*, 1: 3–7.

Pines, M. (1979) Therapeutic communities in teaching hospitals. In: *Therapeutic Communities – Reflections and Progress* (eds R.D. Hinshelwood & N. Manning), Chapter 3. London: Routledge and Kegan Paul.

Pringle, P. (1998) A model of psychosocial care for severe personality disorder. *Nursing Times*, 94 (20): 53–6.

Pringle, P. (1999) *Time limited psychosocial intervention with patients with severe personality disorder following shorter in-patient stay*. Outreach nurse final 3-year research report to North Thames Research and Development, London.

Pringle, P. & Chiesa, M. (2001) From the therapeutic community to the community: developing an outreach psychosocial nursing service for severe personality disorders. *Therapeutic Communities*, 22 (3): 215–32.

Rayner, E. (1986) *Human Development*. London: Allen and Unwin.

Roberts, V. (1994) The self assigned impossible task. In: *The Unconscious at Work* (eds A. Obholzer & V. Roberts), Chapter 12. London: Routledge.

Robinson, S. (1994) Life after death. *Therapeutic Communities*, 15 (2): pp. 77–86.

Rustin, M. (2001) Research evidence and psychotherapy. In: *Evidence in the Psychological Therapies* (eds C. Mace, S. Moorey & B. Roberts). London: Brunner-Routledge.

Sainsbury Centre for Mental Health (2000) *Capabilities of the Modern Mental Health Practitioner: A Model of Lists and Competencies*. Draft consultation Document. London: Sainsbury Centre for Mental Health.

Salzberger-Wittenberg, I. (1970) *Psychoanalytic Insights and Relationships*. London: Routledge.

Salzberger-Wittenberg, I., Henry, G. & Osbourne, E. (1983) *The Emotional Experience of Learning and Teaching*. London: Routledge and Kegan Paul.

Schroder, P.J. (1985) Recognising transference and countertransference. *Journal of Psychosocial Nursing*, 23 (2): pp. 21–6.

Siegler, M. & Osmond, H. (1976) *Models of Madness, Models of Medicine*. New York: Macmillan.

Simpson, A. (1998) Mary's story. In: *Face to Face with Distress: The Professional Use of Self in Psychosocial Care* (eds E. Barnes, P. Griffiths, J. Ord & D. Wells), Chapter 8. Oxford: Butterworth Heinemann.

Simpson, E.A. (1994) Psychological and family centred nursing in the local community. *Journal of Psychiatric and Mental Health Nursing*, 2, 129–30.

Stanton, A. & Schwartz, M. (1954) *The Mental Hospital*. New York: Basic Books.

Stevenson, C. (1996) The tao, social constructionism and psychiatric nursing practice and research. *Journal of Psychiatric and Mental Health Nursing*, 3: 217–24.

Streeck, U. (1997) Supervision in mental health teams and institutions. In: *Supervision and its Vicissitudes* (eds B. Martindale, M. Morner, M.E.C. Rodriquez & J. Vidit), Chapter 4. London: Karnac Books.

Teising, M. (2000) 'Sister, I am going crazy, help me': psychodynamic-orientated care in psychotic patients in inpatient treatment. *Journal of Psychiatric and Mental Health Care*, 7: 449–54.

Tilley, S. (ed.) (1997) *The Mental Health Nurse: Views of Practice and Education*. Edinburgh: Blackwell Science.

Tonnesman, M. (1979) Containing stress in professional work: the human encounter in the caring professions. *Social Work Services Magazine* (DHSS), 21: 34–41.

Trent, D.R. (1992) Breaking the single continuum. In: *Promotion of Mental Health* (ed. D.R. Trent), Vol. 1, pp. 117–26. Aldershot: Avebury.

Trist, E. & Murray, H. (eds) (1990) *The Social Engagement of Social Science. Volume 1: The Socio-Psychological Perspective*. London: Free Association Books.

UKCC (2000) *The Nursing and Midwifery and Health Visiting Contribution to the Continuing Care of People with Mental Health Problems: A Review and UKCC Action Plan*. London: UKCC.

UKCC (2001) *Fitness for Practice. The Report of the UKCC's Post-Commission Development Group*. London: UKCC.

Waddell, D. (1955) Psychology as applied to nursing. A series of notes for tutors and others concerned in the training of student nurses. *Nursing Times*, September 1954–March 1955: 959–60.

Waddell, D. (1968) Change of approach. In: *Psychosocial Nursing: Studies from the Cassel Hospital* (ed. E. Barnes), Chapter 6. London: Tavistock.

Waddell, M. (1998) *Inside Lives: Psychoanalysis and the Growth of Personality*. London: Duckworth.

Wegner, G.D. & Alexander, R.J. (1999) *Readings in Family Nursing*. Philadelphia: Lippincott.

Wells, D., Clifford, D., Rutter, M. & Selby, J. (2000) *Caring for Sexuality in Health and Illness*. London: Churchill Livingstone.

Whyte, D. (ed.) (1997) *Explorations in Family Nursing*. London: Routledge.

Winnicott, W. (1965) The mentally ill in your caseload. In: *The Maturational Processes and the Facilitating Environment*, Chapter 20. London: Hogarth Press.

Winnicott, W. (1971) *Playing and Reality*. London: Tavistock.

Winship, G. (1995a) Nursing and psychoanalysis – uneasy alliances. *Psychoanalytic Psychotherapy*, 9 (3): 289–99.

Winship, G. (1995b) The unconscious impact of caring for acutely disturbed patients. A perspective for supervision. *Journal of Psychiatric and Mental Health Nursing*, 2: 227–33.

Winship, G. (1998) Intensive psychiatric care nursing – psychoanalytic perspectives. *Journal of Psychiatric and Mental Health Nursing*, 5: 1–5.

Winship, G., Harnimann, B., Burling, S. & Courtney, J. (1995) Understanding countertransference and object relations in the process of nursing drug dependant patients. *Psychoanalytic Psychotherapy*, 9 (2): 195–207.

Woodhouse, D. & Pengelly, P. (1991) *Anxiety and the Dynamics of Collaboration*. Aberdeen: Aberdeen University Press.

Wright, H. (1989) *Group Work: Perspectives and Practice*. London: Scutari Press.

Wright, H. (1991) The patient, the nurse, his life and her mother: psychodynamic influences in nurse education and practice. *Psychoanalytic Psychotherapy*, 5 (2): 139–49.

Wright, H. (1996) Psychodynamic nursing: the cultural matrix. Key note paper given at the *Association for Psycho Analytic Psychotherapy Conference, The Culture of Nursing: Psychoanalytic Perspectives*, nurses sub-section, October.

Wright, H. & Giddy, M. (eds) (1993) *Mental Health Nursing: From First Principles to Professional Practice*. Oxford: Chapman Hall.

Wright, L.M. & Leahey, M. (2000) *Nurses and Families: A Guide to Family Assessment and Intervention*, 3rd edn. Philadelphia, F.A. Davis.

Chapter 5

Mental Health Nursing: Principles in Practice

Alexander McMurdo Carson

> But the story-teller has a peculiarly directive influence over us . . . He is able to guide the current of our emotions, to dam it up in one direction and make it flow in another. (Freud, cited in Rieff 1965)

Introduction

This chapter will examine the production of a syllabus for the education and training of registered mental health nurses in a college of higher education. This college is situated in a large town surrounded by a rural mix of small- and medium-sized villages. Originally, the college was the local technical college or 'tech', but it has grown in recent years and now offers both undergraduate and postgraduate courses. The college has aspirations, in the longer term, to become a university. In a nursing context, the college offers undergraduate (diploma) programmes in adult nursing, mental health nursing and children's nursing. The nursing department was originally the local school of nursing but has relocated to higher education following the Project 2000 reforms in nurse education. The department has been a part of the college of higher education for over 10 years. The department has contracts with the English National Board for Nursing, to educate and train a specified number of registered nurses every year. The Nursing and Midwifery Council (NMC) reviews the quality of the educational provision at least yearly and continuance of the contract depends on a positive outcome of the review. Equally, the production of registered nurses is of interest to local Health Trusts, as they need to keep their workforce numbers topped up.

In the last few years, difficulties between nurse education and Health Trusts have led to a review of the education of nurses, leading to the *Fitness for Practice* report (UKCC 1999). This will lead to major changes in the preparation of registered nurses. However, the scheme of education and training that will be examined in this chapter is a 'Project 2000' model. The education and training of registered nurses, using the Project 2000 structure, involves dividing the syllabus into a generic Common Foundation Programme (CFP), which is half of the total course, and a specific Branch Programme, focusing on the production of either registered general nurses, registered children's nurses or registered mental health nurses.

In this chapter, we focus on the Branch Programme that leads to the successful students being awarded the title of registered mental nurse (RMN). Part of the knowledge students are assumed to bring to the Branch Programme is that they 'know' that there are different types of registered nurses and that they are aiming to qualify as RMNs. The relationships between staff in the college, the National Boards, local Health Trusts and students all have some influence on the construction of the nursing curriculum. As well as the more formal 'knowledge' that is part of the contents of the curriculum, part of this particular field of knowledge involves knowing one's way around the political, economic and professional contexts in which the curriculum is situated. A careful analysis of departmental documentation would reveal these various influences and contexts. However, in this chapter I want to review the more formal contents of one particular scheme of training, the Mental Health Branch Programme. While pointing out some of the difficulties with this particular corner of the field of knowledge that is mental health nursing, I also want to articulate one or two things that are missing from the field. Before doing any of this, I think that it is important to be clear about what a review is.

Principles in practice

A review of anything, whether literature, text or practice, inevitably changes what was originally there. To review something is to look again at it; this process involves a degree of reflectiveness or thought and choice. As in ordinary life, reviewing can help us to see something that we perhaps did not see the first time. For instance, I buy a pair of shoes because I like the style or the colour. However, while wearing them I meet a friend who congratulates me on wearing such 'trendy' footwear and for being so brave. Now when I look again at my shoes I see that I have been acting foolishly, trying to appear young and that, after all, fluorescent blue does not really match any of my other clothes. A review involves a change in perspective and this necessarily changes what was there before. Originally, my shoes seemed very nice but they now seem foolish. In reviewing my original choice, I see that it was mistaken and I hand the shoes in to a charity shop. While this kind of review, based on personal preferences, is the kind of practice that we all have in common, it is nothing more than changing one's mind. Although this is normally a good enough rationale in ordinary life, something more is required in proposing to review someone else's work. This chapter, as a review, will suggest things that the original writers of this particular curriculum perhaps did not see. In reviewing a syllabus for the education and training of mental health nurses, a *responsible* review has to provide a rationale that is more than simply a change of mind. An implicit assumption of this review is that it provides a *better*, rather than simply a different, view of what is there. So this chapter, as well as simply looking again at an educational programme, will also provide an explicit justification for its assertion that this new view is better and more reflective than the original.

A decisive factor in the choice of keeping or getting rid of the shoes was the view I have of myself. Equally, a significant factor that could help to arbitrate between the original syllabus and this review would be a view that mental health nursing has of itself. Few, I think, would disagree with the idea that mental health nursing is a method of helping people who suffer from a disabling condition. Wherever and whenever it is practised mental health nursing is always about helping people who are suffering from a particular disabling condition called mental illness. What constitutes mental illness has been and still is a matter of dispute, but what is not in dispute is that mental health nursing, like all other branches of nursing, is about the relief of suffering. A criterion or standard that could help to guide our review and that we could expect to find in the original syllabus would be this ethic of help. We would expect to see this ethic of help articulated in all practices that are concerned with mental health nursing, whether the practices are situated in clinical, educational or institutional contexts. Much of the time this standard is implicit in practice, buried and out of sight. Yet it provides the foundations and the rationale for all of the practices that are associated with mental health nursing. In a modern context this standard might be referred to as a 'core' value. It would be true to say that without this core value, of helping people who suffer a disabling condition, the practice is not mental health nursing. This ethical standard or value would be what Blum and McHugh (1985) call a 'principle'. While this review will be an excavation of a particular practice, namely producing an educational programme, it could be seen as a principled review in that it is guided by an explicit standard. Before saying more about the programme itself, it might be useful to say a little about this particular standard or principle.

As Blum and McHugh use the term, a principle is the *determinant sense of value* of any practice. In nursing, we often think of principles as abstract rules or standards that should be applied in all situations. For instance the NMC issues standards or principles for nursing practice in a 'Code of Professional Conduct'. This code includes notions such as respect for patients and not doing patients any harm. However, because of their abstractness, they do not necessarily help individual nurses in particular situations, as they are not sensitive enough to particular circumstances. These standards or principles are formulated externally from all practices, although their intention is that they can be meaningfully applied in all practices and circumstances. However, a standard such as not harming a patient does not automatically help or provide sufficient pre-guaranteed guidance to a nurse who is dealing with a patient who has a terminal illness and a chest infection. Should antibiotics be given? Will it improve the quality of the patient's life? Will it do more harm than good? These practical considerations are the everyday concerns of professional practice. Abstract principles, though necessary, help in a very limited way. By contrast, Blum and McHugh define principles as standards that are embedded in each particular practice rather than as abstract rules that should be applied, in a more or less meaningful way, to all practices.

Blum and McHugh also distinguish their notion of principles from Wittgenstein's insight that we should think of practices as language games, since they are articulated or 'made' within language (Blum and McHugh 1985). Like any game, each practice is constructed from and governed by rules; achieving competence in any practice is about knowing the rules that constitute or make the practice what it is or claims to be. For instance, buying shoes is a practice that requires a knowledge and competent use of a series of rules. To buy shoes we need to know what 'buying' is, what shoes are and so on and then we need to be able to do 'buying shoes'. While we can, as competent adults, competently buy shoes, the rules that we use in constructing the practice of buying shoes are implicit in the practice. Blum and McHugh develop this notion of rules by pointing out that seeing practices as solely constituted by rules would make each practice the equivalent of all other practices; all are constituted by rules. In their major work *Self-Reflection in the Arts and Sciences* (Blum and McHugh 1985), they begin by assuming that some of our practices are more important or valuable than others. Buying shoes is not as significant or valuable a practice as mental health nursing. While buying shoes might give me satisfaction or pleasure, mental health nursing amounts to something more significant than personal satisfaction. Blum and McHugh have developed an analytical method, which they call self-reflection, which is designed both to identify the rules that are used to construct a practice and to evaluate these rules against the claim that the practice implicitly makes about itself. They assume that all practices aim for some good or principle that justifies the practice. Their reflective method is a way of measuring the practice's claims about itself and the practice itself. They want to distinguish between the rules that give the practice its structure and the principle that gives the practice its significance or determinant sense of value. They suggest that, in examining the text or any other practice, this principle should be seen in the practice. Self-reflection is a review or looking again at the practice to see if the practice's claims to be significant are realized in the practice. As such, self-reflection begins with the practice rather than developing abstract or external principles to measure the practice against. Their method is a critical dialogue or conversation between the practice and the significance or good that the practice claims for itself. Unlike other conventional critical methods, Blum and McHugh want to give the practices they examine as good a hearing or reading as the practice can possibly bear. However, while the practice proposes to be a good practice, their method of self-reflection can show that the practice can actually fail to deliver on its proposal.

In the introduction to this chapter, helping people who suffer from a disabling condition was identified as a good that mental health nursing aims for. In examining this particular practice, the writing of a curriculum for mental health nursing, we can assume that the curriculum also proposes itself as being able to help people who suffer from a disabling condition. The rest of the chapter will be the development of a dialogue between the practice or curriculum and the good or principle that it is proposing for itself. In reviewing a practice such as formulating a syllabus for the education and training of mental health nurses, we should see 'evidence' of this principle in practice. This review will be guided by this principle as it looks again at the particular syllabus as a social practice. For convenience, the syllabus is divided into two areas, a theory section and a practice section. The theory section focuses on the underlying rationale, philosophy and knowledge of this particular syllabus. The practice components focus on the practical methods of achieving the theoretical aims.

Mental health nursing: theory

The scheme of training or syllabus produced in this college is a Branch Programme in mental health nursing. The programme is arranged under eight broad headings:

- Course Details
- Financial Arrangements
- Course Management
- Course Curriculum
- Course Content, Structure and Organization
- Practical Experience
- Assessment of Competence
- Methods of Internal Evaluation of the Course

Course details include the name and length of the course and selection procedures. Financial matters include course fees and budgetary details. The course management section is a membership list with terms of reference. As a percentage of the documents, these three sections amount to less than 10% of the total. The overwhelming emphasis (over 90%) in this programme is on knowledge of educational methods as well as other discrete forms of knowledge. This is hardly surprising in documents that have to tell a convincing story about educational competence. The final three sections account for less than 5% of the total, so the majority of the documentation is focused around the fourth and fifth sections. These two sections, which account for 85% of the total, I will designate the theory and practice sections. Section 4 (the theory) deals with the course curriculum including the course philosophy, rationale and the curricular model used. Section 5 (the practice) outlines the methods that will be used and the specialized knowledge that will be provided to enact the course philosophy. Before discussing the practical knowledge that is a part of the programme, I want to look at the theory of the course and measure it against our ethic of help.

The 'Philosophy' that begins the curricular documents states that mental health nursing is grounded in a 'belief in the holistic nature of people and the right of every individual to equal respect'. Here, the curriculum philosophy defines both mental health nursing and its relationships to clients as a practice that respects clients as whole people, worthy of respect. In terms of our principle of always helping people, this is evidence that helps to fill in a picture of what mental health nurses should do if they want to practise in a principled way. Helping people who suffer a disabling condition means treating clients as whole people, worthy of respect. We could argue that help and respect were mutually constitutive concepts in that one could not be what it is without the other. Could we really be helping a client if we did not treat that person with respect or tried to degrade him or her? An essential part of this ethic of help is that nurses in a mental health context first of all respect their clients as whole people. While respect for the whole person is consistent with an ethic of help, it is also consistent with our societal norm of respect for persons. Charles Taylor (1992) sees modern life as essentially constituted by a number of universal values or 'hyper goods'. These hyper goods are what Taylor thinks essentially define modern life. Taylor thinks that respect for persons, by virtue of their being persons, is one of these modern hyper goods. He points out that no country now does not subscribe to the idea that people, as persons, are due respect. Even the worst criminals/terrorists are universally acknowledged as having the right to be treated in a dignified way. The current debate over the treatment of al-Qaida prisoners in a military detention center in Cuba is not about whether they *should* be treated with respect but whether they *are* being treated in a way that maintains their dignity as human beings. Even after the events of 11 September it will be difficult for this universal value to be challenged theoretically. This is not to say that some practices cannot fail to reach this standard, but it seems unlikely that anyone could make a valid claim that some human beings were not entitled to respect. This curriculum, like society as a whole, acknowledges this ethic of respect and situates it within mental health nursing.

This particular corner of the field of knowledge is circumscribed by a moral boundary or ethical framework in the shape of an ethics of treating people as whole persons who are worthy of respect. The philosophy expressed in the curriculum demonstrates that mental health nursing helps people who suffer a disabling condition by first of all treating them as whole people, worthy of respect. We can begin to fill in some of the other features of the field such as the various skills, techniques and knowledge required in this particular context. I have referred to this latter part of the curriculum as the more 'practical' part of the curriculum as it more specifically aims at clinical practice. This is not to say that producing a curriculum and caring for a client with a mental health problem are not both social practices. The conventional view has been to talk about issues such as the 'theory–practice' gap. The *Fitness for Practice* report alluded to earlier, was based on the assumption that we really could make a distinction between theory, as activities that go on in educational institutions, and practice, as activities that are situated in clinical contexts. I do not want to go into the issue here, but I think that the distinction conventionally made is a gloss on how things really are. All practices are examples of theorizing and all theorizings are examples of social practices. The idea that we could neatly separate theory and practice would mean that we literally could have a theory-free practice. What would it look like? While 'practical' people often talk as if they had no theory to orient to, their minimalist practice would still need some theoretical orientation to be recognized as something other than random movement. Imagine asking a mental health nurse what she or he was doing? Without some theoretical underpinnings the nurse would at best claim that he or she was simply moving. By and large, people see and describe what they are doing as something more than movement and for this they need a theoretical explanation such as 'I'm waiting for a bus' or 'I'm talking to this client'. These accounts of our practices assume a theory of public transport, timetables, social etiquette, health services, professions, clients and so on. The distinction that is often made between theory and practice in nursing is based on a convention or agreement rather than on the way things really are. Nevertheless I will use practice as it is defined in the curriculum, as activities that go on in clinical contexts. In the next section, we can examine some of the practical skills that are needed for clinical practice.

Mental health nursing: practice

The rest of the curriculum is more explicitly devoted to contributing to fitting students for future practice as registered nurses. The methods chosen to meet this purpose include an equal mix of college work, the 'theory' part of the programme, and clinical experience, the 'practice' component. Students who enter the programme are recognized as entering the programme with a history rather than as blank pages that need to be filled in. The programme aims to enhance development based on each student's particular life experiences by equipping them with 'the knowledge and understanding, skills, values and beliefs relevant in the context of mental health'. Mental health nursing is defined as a 'human activity' that allows professionals to 'intellectually intervene' in response to the 'behavioural, emotional, cognitive and spiritual problems' of clients.

This curriculum provides a structure for learning that is pyramidal and progressive. It is arranged around the educational taxonomies of cognitive, affective and psychomotor skills. Cognitively, students on the programme move from being able to describe and explain things to being critical and analytical thinkers. The programme is divided into four clear blocks:

- Mental health care in society
- Mental health care in group settings
- Mental health care with individual clients
- Preparation for practice.

Students are progressed from larger contexts to smaller ones, from experiencing mental health nursing in larger contexts to working with individual clients. The formal knowledge that is prescribed for these experiences includes nursing theory and practice, the biological and behavioural sciences and professional issues. It is very similar to a curriculum generated for adult nursing. In Biology, the focus is on ageing, neurological science, endocrine disorders and stress. This section is heavily influenced by a medical perspective on mental illness, with its emphasis on mental illness as an organic disorder. In the section on Law and Ethics, the emphasis is on legal aspects of mental health nursing. The formal knowledge part of the curriculum is designed clearly as 'theory', which provides prescriptions that can be tried out in the student's practice placements. Explicitly, the programme aims at producing a *'competent autonomous practitioner'*, organized around the student progressing from being a *knowledgeable observer* through being a *supervised participant* to being *therapeutically involved*. Competence is organized around these three key stages of development. The ability to be therapeutically involved is a measure of the competence of an autonomous practitioner and as such is a standard that all successful students have to reach.

The rationale for arranging the students' clinical experiences from larger contexts to working with individual clients and the development of a competent practitioner is not explicitly outlined in the documents. These practice placements are seen as the contexts in which theory comes face-to-face with clinical reality. The curriculum and practice placements combine to produce an educational route from observer to competent practitioner. In this curriculum there is a very close relationship between therapeutic involvement and clinical competence. The assertion in the documents is that competence can be measured against a student's ability to be 'therapeutically involved'. In the next section, I want to look more closely at this relationship.

The production of competence

The wider context in which mental health nursing operates is the health care system. The *Fitness for Practice* report (UKCC 1999) identified a problem with the competence of newly qualified nurses. In medicine, the competence of doctors has been under attack, following the Bristol heart surgery scandal and the Harold Shipman affair. Indeed, the competence of the people who supervise and certify the competence of doctors is the subject of current debate. There is a generalized public feeling that there should be more lay involvement in the regulation of professional competence. The structure of the United Kingdom Central Council for Nursing, Midwifery and Health Visiting (UKCC), now the Nursing and Midwifery Council (NMC), reflects this imperative for more public involvement. Political announcements and publications (NHS Wales 2001) emphasize the need for greater public participation in the health care system. It is no longer tenable to smugly reassure the public that matters relating to the competence of health care professionals can be left to internal, professional regulation. As a result of these changes, definitions of competence may begin to alter to reflect increasing public influence. I think that currently under-rated values such as empathy, openness and treating patients as whole people will assume greater influence in definitions of competence. However, this particular syllabus equates competence with the ability to be therapeutically involved with clients and it is this notion of therapeutic involvement that I want to focus on now.

In an account of psychiatric nursing, Tilley (1995) described certain influences that currently available models of psychiatric nursing share. As well as being influenced by a version of scientific rationality, Tilley states that they are situated within a:

discourse of care and/or therapy, linked with a discourse on inter-professional distinctions and the need for nurses to establish their domains of competence *vis à vis* psychiatrists and social workers. (Tilley 1995: 129)

In accounting for what they do, according to Tilley, psychiatric nurses use a number of different language games as resources in defining themselves and their relationships with other professionals. These language games are used internally within the field of psychiatric nursing, as nurses account to their colleagues for what they are doing. Externally, these language games are used to ward off potential transgressors into their field, such as psychiatrists, non-psychiatric nurses and social workers.

This particular curriculum shares certain language games with other nurses who care for adults or children. Biology, sociology and psychology are examples of common language games that the curriculum proposes to teach students so that the students can develop awareness 'of the process of human behaviour as a fundamental pre-requisite of intellectual intervention'. While there is a good argument that could be made that an awareness of the 'process of human behaviour' would be required in any nursing syllabus, the notion of therapeutic involvement seems to be a language game that is distinctive to mental health nursing, as both Tilley and the curriculum suggest. Moreover, Tilley asserts that this discourse is partly organized around a practical model of scientific rationality, while the curriculum suggests a similar model of practice, intellectual intervention. There is often assumed to be a close affinity between the notion of professionalism, intellectual intervention and scientific rationality. Images of the clinical, objective approach to clients' problems are still seen as a possible model of professional practice. Most nurses, irrespective of their distinctive clinical specialisms, share this particular part of the field of knowledge. Therapeutic intervention, by contrast, is often seen as a softer, more client-centered approach to problems. Both Tilley and this particular curriculum suggest that therapeutic involvement is a distinctive language game that psychiatric nurses use in defining themselves and their particular claims to competence. This is a crucial issue, as therapy seems to be an important boundary marker for psychiatric nurses. Interestingly, Tilley asserts that the relationship between care and therapy is an 'and/or' relationship and this assumes that care and therapy are different concepts, although they are often combined in practice. I think that this is a gloss on how things really are in psychiatric nursing. However, before looking at the relationship between care and therapy, we need to look at what therapy means to psychiatric nurses.

Therapeutic involvement, according to Wright (1997), is a way nurses mediate both internal and external dangers that may appear in the nurse–client relationship, particularly dangers that may emanate from the emotions. According to Wright, therapeutic involvement can help the mental health nurse both manage his or her own emotional feelings and avert the possibility of being overwhelmed by the client's emotions and distress. Many of the clients encountered by psychiatric nurses have emotional difficulties that are overwhelming them and could potentially overwhelm the nurse; therapies are methods for deflecting that danger. The problem, as perceived by Wright and others in this field, is that working with mentally ill people can be hazardous if a nurse gets too close either to the client or to his or her own emotions. Therapeutic involvement is a practical method for allowing a mental health nurse to maintain some control over his or her emotions and/or maintain some control over the client's emotional condition. On the surface it looks like a more person-centered approach, a softer more subjective practice, but in reality, it shares some common features with other practices such as intellectual intervention and scientific rationality. All are practices that are linked by ideas of control and the possible elimination of emotions from practice. Scientific rationality and intellectual intervention are language games that are partly constituted by a detached, dispassionate approach. In adopting these language games, this particular curriculum and psychiatric nursing in general seem to be excluding emotional knowledge from their field of knowledge. Both the emotional life of the client and the emotional life of the nurse are excluded from the psychiatric nurse–client relationship. Before saying something relating to the field of knowledge, I want to say something about two main problems arising with this model of practice. The first issue relates to power and control, while the more serious relates to matters of competency.

In terms of control and power, to prescribe an encounter between a psychiatric nurse and a client as a therapeutic intervention, in advance of actually meeting a client, is to prescribe a context in advance of a 'real' situation. In the earlier example of buying a pair of shoes, there was more than one way to 'see' these shoes: nice or foolish. In an encounter between a psychiatric nurse and a client, there is a choice of at least two points of view. To prescribe a situation in advance as a 'therapeutic' encounter is to presume to 'know' something about the client and his or her situation. However, at a practical level, this knowledge could be an obstruction to understanding the client's view of the situation. Therapeutic intervention presumes to know that all clients require some form of therapy. Many of the clients that psychiatric nurses encounter may well require therapy, but not *all* of them. Some clients may have practical problems, some might be looking for a friend or looking for attention or may have nothing wrong with them; therapy is not *always* a solution to clients' problems. In terms of the measurement of competence, the ability to be therapeutically involved cannot be a standard or principle, as it would look like psychiatric nurses were sometimes practising incompetently if they found themselves in situations with clients where no therapy was appropriate. Perhaps psychiatric nurses would define themselves as essentially a 'therapeutic' profession. Here, Wright's rationale for therapy as a protection from internal (the nurse's) and external (the client's) emotions could be used as a justification for this model of psychiatric nursing and its field of knowledge. However, a more serious difficulty arises. This relates to the psychiatric nurse's philosophical aim of treating clients as whole people, worthy of respect.

Both psychiatric nurses and their clients have emotional lives that are a part of who they are as whole persons. While the so-called drama queen represents an exaggerated image of the emotional life, there is no doubt that most people consider the emotions as an essential attribute or characteristic of being human. Part of modern life is about getting 'in touch' with our inner selves, our feelings and emotions. Nowadays, the traditional British 'stiff upper lip' is seen as a repressed form of humanity, an unhealthy attitude to life. The cool professionalism and clear-sightedness of Sherlock Holmes was attributed to his ability to put aside his emotions, while his friend and biographer, Dr Watson, the incompetent bumbler, brought a human touch to the stories by getting too close to the clients and cases; indeed, he marries one of Holmes' clients. However, the cost of Holmes' brilliance as a detective was his narrowness as a human being. Without our emotions we are not fully whole human beings. The picture of Holmes, with his solitary pleasures of cocaine and the violin, produces pity in the reader as we see that there is a tremendous cost in developing too narrowly as a person. Emotions are not thought of, particularly today, as something that we can take or leave but as something that are an essential part of who we are as persons. We often evaluate situations on the basis of their 'feel' and we often hear people saying that they just feel something 'in their water' or have a 'gut' feeling about something or someone. Holmes' model of practice, screening out the emotional, helped him to solve 'interesting' problems. He never gets to see the person with the problem and so he usually solves the problem.

Although Sherlock Holmes was interested in solving crime rather than giving therapy, his practice and mental health nursing, as specified in the curriculum, are similar. Both fail to see the whole person, as both are premised on ruling out the emotions as distractions or dangers. Moreover, both practices impose conditions in advance of involvement with clients, by specifying what kind of involvement, whether scientific or intellectual intervention or therapeutic involvement; these conditions effectively rule out seeing clients as whole people. In some ways, Sherlock Holmes has clients who are more interested in solving a crime than in being treated holistically. This is not the case with psychiatric nursing, as articulated in this particular curriculum, which defines itself as a practice that treats clients as whole people, worthy of respect. A psychiatric nurse who approached clients with therapeutic involvement as a prescription or standard would be failing to practise in what could be called a 'principled' way. This prescription is inconsistent with the principle, articulated at the beginning of the curriculum, clients as whole people that nurses should treat. Perhaps there are times when a certain emotional detachment would be necessary when dealing with clients with mental health problems. However, the curriculum specifies that competent mental health nurses are *always* therapeutically involved, and this involves limiting or abolishing any emotional content in nurse–client encounters.

This issue goes to the heart of what is required in someone who aspires to be a competent mental health practitioner. Real situations or encounters between psychiatric nurses and clients involve relationship between whole people; that is, people, like nurses and clients, who are partly constituted by their emotions. The client, produced in this curriculum, is still the 'bio-psycho-social' agent of much nursing theory (Roper *et al.* 1990). In this respect, the curriculum is no different from most other nursing curricula. It contains universal prescriptions for practice, in this case 'therapeutic involvement'; prescriptions that need to be competently applied in practice. Mental health practice would be about assuming that all clients needed a therapeutic relationship and thus therapeutic involvement would be less of a professional choice and more of a professional obligation. As such it is always a part of practice and applies in *all* situations. However, this practical method is inconsistent with a curriculum that claims to respect clients as whole people and a profession that is situated within an ethic of helping people who suffer from a disabling condition. Not all clients may need or be helped by therapy; it might even do some harm to some people. The controversies over various therapies, in areas such as repressed memories or sexual abuse, should make us think more about their value. However, this particular curriculum provides no way of evaluating individual clients' needs for therapy; this means that, in practice, a psychiatric nurse has no way of 'knowing' whether a therapeutic involvement is necessarily helping his or her client. This is not to say that the use of therapeutic involvement is not a valuable part of practice or of the field of psychiatric nursing knowledge. As I have already indicated, therapeutic involvement is sometimes necessary and so it remains a possible choice of method for psychiatric nurses.

In terms of the competent mental health nurse, therapeutic involvement leaves out too much of what is really going on in encounters with whole people. Relating to clients therapeutically, as a universal method, is relating to clients from a distance. It produces an image of mental illness as a danger that psychiatric nurses need protection from. In these universalized therapeutic encounters, clients and psychiatric nurses are defined narrowly rather than as the whole people they really are.

In this review of a particular curriculum, defining therapeutic involvement as a standard for practice means sometimes practising in an unprincipled way. Moreover, this particular curriculum excludes emotional knowledge from the field of mental health nursing. In the next section, I want to suggest a practical method that could help psychiatric nurses to treat their clients as whole people; but as part of this would involve taking knowledge of clients' emotions more seriously, I will first of all say something about this.

The whole story

We could think of respect for clients as whole people as a principle that *always* animates psychiatric nursing practice. By contrast, therapeutic involvement is more like a rule that is *sometimes* necessary in practice. A principle such as respect still leaves room for the exercise of a strong model of professional judgment. If a practitioner in mental health nursing always saw each situation as a case for therapeutic involvement, professional judgment would be limited to deciding which particular therapy was appropriate rather than the more critical question of whether any therapy was required. This weak model of decision-making seems to discount the experience, intuition and tacit knowledge of mental health nurses. It also raises the question of how autonomous this practitioner really is. Part of professional judgment is choosing which particular interventions, or whether any interventions, are thought to help clients. A principle such as treating clients as whole people does not impede professional judgment, but enhances it. Now the question faced by practitioners is explicitly one of expanding their field of knowledge to develop methods or practices that are consistent with treating clients as whole persons, worthy of respect. In the context of this book, I want to suggest two particular areas of knowledge that mental health nursing needs to cultivate and claim, if it is to define itself more clearly as a distinctive field of knowledge.

Each of us has an emotional life, without which we would not be who we are. So emotions are constitutive of who we are as human beings. To try to do away with our emotions would diminish us as people and so I think that mental health nursing should grasp this particular nettle. I also think that we should not be thinking simply of developing new techniques for controlling the emotions. Emotions are good and bad, healthy and unhealthy, shallow and deep. They are certainly too complex to simply make up a recipe for practice that would cover all clients. The emotions, in particular, need not be viewed as impediments to psychiatric nursing knowledge; they can instead be seen as part of the embodied knowledge of both clients and mental health nurses. Martha Nussbaum, in *The Therapy of Desire* (Nussbaum 1994), contends that literature and philosophy can help educate and cultivate our emotional health. She provides a model of holistic practice that does not want to shield us from our own or other people's emotions. She believes that emotions are a necessary part of our self-understandings as whole people. So I think that there is a place in mental health nursing for a fresh approach to the emotions; in particular, Nussbaum's idea that we can educate and cultivate the emotions. Of course, there are other writers who view the emotions as an essential part of human life, but it seems that mental health nursing needs to expand its field of knowledge to include knowledge of the emotions.

Another method that could help psychiatric nurses to treat their clients with respect is listening seriously to the stories that their clients tell. This does not mean that clients' stories should be viewed as 'information' or 'data', to be cut up and fitted to pre-existing frameworks such as models of nursing (Riehl & Roy 1980). While these models have provided a wider choice of assessment to practising nurses, they will inevitably be reductionist. Their attempts to 'fit' the patient into the prescribed assessment framework will necessarily result in failing to see the whole person and this particular person's experience. It seems very unlikely that any single assessment framework, however flexibly applied and interpreted, could fully capture the patient's suffering and hurt. In medicine itself, there has been an increased awareness in the value of a more narrative-based medicine (Greenhalgh & Hurwitz 1999). Greenhalgh & Hurwitz recommend that there should be a revival of interest in narratives, in the teaching and practice of medicine. As they point out, modern medicine lacks:

. . . a metric for existential qualities such as the inner hurt, despair, hope, grief, and moral pain that frequently accompany, and often indeed constitute, the illnesses from which people suffer. (Greenhalgh & Hurwitz 1999: 50)

Equally, in difficult ethical situations, it is contended that doctors can learn from listening to their patients' stories rather than simply proceeding on the basis of scientific, medical knowledge (Hudson Jones 1999). An old story, quoted by Hannah Arendt (Arendt 1989), will illustrate the point. The story is told about a philosopher called Demosthenes. A man once approached Demosthenes and related how terribly he had been beaten. 'But you,' said Demosthenes, 'suffered nothing of what you tell me.' Whereupon the other raised his voice and cried out: **'I suffered nothing?'** 'Now,' said Demosthenes, 'I hear the voice of somebody who was injured and who suffered.' In this example we see that a conversation or story, told in the right way, can reveal the suffering that is often an essential part of any misfortune. A dry recounting of the facts, as originally spoken by Demosthenes' friend, can fail to capture the hurt and suffering involved. In expressing his indignation, his friend revealed the person who was hurt and who had suffered. Methods or practices such as therapeutic involvement hide the person from view and produce a practice that fails to see the client as a person who is suffering.

Conclusion

In reviewing my particular part of the field of knowledge, I have tried to indicate some problems in clearly defining what this field would look like. While the curriculum included knowledge that would be common to most nursing curricula, such as biology, psychology and sociology, it also laid claim to a distinctive form of knowledge or language game that belonged to mental health nurses. However, this claim for distinction was found to go against its claim that it always treated clients in a principled way, as whole persons worthy of respect. This review was a reflection on a particular practice (the construction of a Branch Programme in mental health nursing) that claims to see something that the original writers did not see or were not aware of. Specifying therapeutic involvement as a measure of competence implies a universal prescription for practice that could obstruct mental health nurses proposing to practise in a principled way. I have also tried to show that too great a reliance on therapeutic knowledge could exclude other very valuable forms of knowledge, including knowledge of the emotions. This syllabus was skeptical about emotional knowledge, viewing it as an obstacle to more valuable forms of knowledge such as scientific rational knowledge. This skepticism has wider echoes in the psychiatric nursing literature, which sees emotions as things to be controlled rather than understood. In conclusion I have suggested that the mental health nurse's field of knowledge should include emotional knowledge and narrative knowledge. I am not suggesting that the client's emotions or story should always dominate the encounters, and I want to finish by suggesting how these can help psychiatric nurses in clinical practice as well as just being interesting in their own right.

Elsewhere, I have outlined a method for helping nurses to mediate between their own view of the situation or problem and the client's view of the problem (Carson 2001). By listening seriously to the client's story, the nurse is provided with an opportunity to look again at the situation he or she is involved in. Professional judgment is about making choices between our perspective on how things are and the client's perspective. The narrative method that I describe does not provide ready-made answers to practical problems or choices, but instead tries to develop a way of evaluating both stories. Sometimes the nurse or health care professional might choose the client's point of view rather than his or her own; sometimes it will be the other way around. In the earlier example of the choice of seeing our shoes as foolish or nice, a crucial factor was the view I had of myself. If psychiatric nursing defines itself as essentially concerned with therapeutic knowledge, the nurse's view of the client will be seriously diminished, as clients will all be thought of as problems in need of therapeutic manipulation. Within the field of knowledge, I have suggested that therapy should be a choice rather than a requirement. To return to Tilley's comments about care and/or therapy, one could ask whether it was possible to care for someone whom one did not respect as a whole person. If a psychiatric nurse did make this kind of choice and chose therapy, would he or she really be caring for someone whom he/she failed to respect? Some parts of psychiatric nursing knowledge are more valuable or significant than others. While the use of therapy might be a choice in practice, caring for people by respecting their wholeness is not a choice but a principle that should always be a part of practice and the field of knowledge that is mental health nursing.

I have also suggested that the inclusion of narrative and emotional knowledge could help psychiatric nurses to develop more empathic knowledge of clients as whole people. Unlike therapeutic knowledge, which could be an obstacle to other knowledge, narrative knowledge and an understanding of the emotions could help develop new models of holistic practice as well as newer, more empathic knowledge of individual clients. This new knowledge would enhance practice and help develop mental health nursing and its field of knowledge. If taken seriously this knowledge could help mental health nurses to understand situations a little better by getting closer to the person who really needs their help. To include more empathic, holistic knowledge in the field would help psychiatric nursing to develop a more principled practice.

References

Arendt, H. (1989) *The Human Condition*. Chicago: University of Chicago Press.

Blum, A. & McHugh, P. (1985) *Self-Reflection in the Arts and Sciences*, New Jersey: Humanities Press Atlantic Highlands.

Carson, A.M. (2001) That's another story: narrative methods and ethical practice. *British Journal of Medical Ethics*, 27: 198–202.

Greenhalgh, T. & Hurwitz, B. (1999) Why study narrative? *British Medical Journal*, 318: 48–50.

Jones, A.H. (1999) Narrative in medical ethics. *British Medical Journal*, 318: 253–6.

NHS Wales (2001) *Signposts: A Practical Guide to Public and Patient Involvement in Wales.* London: Office for Public Management.

Nussbaum, M.C. (1994) *The Therapy of Desire: Theory and Practice in Hellenistic Ethics.* New Jersey: Princeton University Press.

Rieff, P. (1965) *Freud: The Mind of the Moralist.* London: Methuen.

Riehl, J.P. & Roy, C. (eds) (1980) *Conceptual Models for Nursing Practice.* New York: Appleton-Century-Crofts,

Roper, N., Logan, W.W. & Tierney, A. (1990) *The Activities of Daily Living.* Edinburgh: Churchill Livingstone.

Taylor, C. (1992) *Sources of the Self. The Making of The Modern Identity.* Cambridge: Cambridge University Press.

Tilley, S. (1995) Accounts, accounting and accountability in psychiatric nursing. In: *Accountability in Nursing Practice* (ed. R. Watson). London: Chapman and Hall.

United Kingdom Central Council for Nursing, Midwifery and Health Visiting (1999) *Fitness for Practice – The UKCC Commission for Nursing and Midwifery Education.* London: UKCC.

Wright, H. (1997) The therapeutic relationship. In: *Mental Health Nursing: From First Principles to Professional Practice* (eds. H. Wright & M. Giddy). Cheltenham: Stanley Thorn.

Chapter 6

Shaping Pre-Registration Mental Health Nursing Education Through User and Carer Involvement in Curriculum Design and Delivery

Susanne Forrest and Hugh Masters

Introduction

The specification for this chapter required us to consider how knowledge of mental health nursing is situated and configured in our institution. In this chapter we provide a reflective account of how our approach to teaching mental health nursing has been shaped over the past six years by our experiences of involving mental health service users and carers in curriculum design and delivery. We first give a description of our involvement work, then progress to discuss how the lessons we learned from this changed our approach to thinking about and teaching mental health nursing, and how this is translated into the curriculum. We then locate our approach to mental health nursing education within our own institution and the wider institutional contexts that also influence pre-registration mental health nursing education.

Background

Napier University, in Edinburgh, is one of Scotland's 'new' Universities and since 1996 has been the largest provider of pre-registration nursing education in Scotland. The Mental Health Team is located within the Faculty of Health and Life Sciences, evolved from a faculty originally established in 1996, when Scottish 'Colleges of Nursing and Midwifery' moved into the Higher Education sector. In Scotland pre-registration nursing education is provided through a contractual agreement between the Scottish Executive and the Higher Education institutions.

During 1996 we commenced the process of designing a new curriculum for the Diploma of Higher Education in Nursing (Mental Health). Part of this process involved consultation with users and carers undertaken in response to policy directives. Perhaps most importantly this consultation was driven primarily by an apathetic response to consultation from service staff and providers. A small research grant from the National Board for Nursing, Midwifery and Health Visiting

101

Scotland (NBS) enabled the consultation to be taken forward as a development project. The initial project had two main aims. The first aim was to elicit users' views about the knowledge, skills and attributes they considered mental health nurses should possess. Second, the research began to explore strategies whereby users and carers could be involved in ongoing curriculum design and delivery. This first phase of our involvement work is detailed in Forrest *et al.* (1998, 2000).

With the continuing support of the NBS a second phase of the project evolved. This had the broad aim of devising a strategy for user and carer involvement in the pre-registration curriculum and concurrently evaluated the strategy development process. The strategy development and evaluation process involved joint project working between academic team members, mental health students, mental health service users and carers. In keeping with recommendations made in Forrest *et al.* (1998), user and carer representatives for the project were recruited via user- and carer-led organisations. The lecturers involved in the initial phase of the project also acted as project members in the second phase (both authors of this chapter took part in both phases). Student members were recruited from two cohorts of students who were then undertaking their pre-registration programme.

A more detailed account of the structures and processes of the strategy development and evaluation is provided in Risk *et al.* (2000). In summary, the project involved establishing a Project Management Group which undertook the initial project planning; and two sub-groups, the 'Strategy Development Group' and the 'Project Evaluation Group'. Both sub-groups contained service uses, carers, students and lecturers, with lecturers comprising fewer than half of the membership. The Strategy Development Group's task was to collect data and eventually write the 'Strategy for Involvement', reported in Risk *et al.* (2000). This was informed through various activities including study tours, internet searching, users and carers observing classes, and meetings between users, carers, the wider mental health teaching team and students.

Concurrently the Project Evaluation Group designed and conducted a research project that evaluated the strategy development process, taking account of the experiences of project members, as well as considering views from a wider group of managers and educationalists within and outwith the Faculty. The findings from the evaluation are discussed in Risk *et al.* (2000) and Masters *et al.* (2002).

Involvement as a knowledge base for pre-registration mental health nursing education

It is useful to start with what knowledge base we drew on prior to commencing our journey through user and carer involvement. Perhaps in common with many mental health nursing education departments now located in other 'new' Universities in Scotland (evolved out of the former Colleges of Nursing), we cannot offer an historical overview that lays claim to a unique and special institutional body of knowledge about mental health nursing. Research development in our own team is in its infancy and 'knowledge' has tended to be 'borrowed' and adapted from other fields such as psychology, sociology and psychiatry. Like others working in mental health education, we faced (and still face) constant external drives to produce curricula that respond to the 'push and pull' of the many, and sometimes conflicting, policy, service and academic agendas. Caught up in this we have historically gone through various curriculum developments, mainly driven by the statutory requirements of professional bodies such as the UKCC and NBS[1] and service agendas.

Where we started from in relation to thinking and teaching about mental health nursing is probably best conceptualised as a 'traditional' approach. By 'traditional' we mean teaching a curriculum likely to be fairly similar, in terms of philosophy, content and approach, to other Project 2000 pre-registration mental health nursing courses delivered in comparable institutions. What we have started to move towards now goes beyond the promotion of user and carer involvement in the curriculum, as originally outlined in our 'Strategy for Involvement', and is best described as a 'user- and carer-informed' approach. Table 6.1 attempts to summarise the differences between the two approaches.

We will now describe how our work with users and carers served to help us begin to construct this approach to mental health nursing education. In doing this we draw on findings from the involvement projects and also on our personal experiences of the process of involvement.

The shift in approach

The starting point in our shift of approach was the findings from our first project which aimed to elicit users' and carers' views about what they perceived as the desired knowledge, skills and attitudes mental health nurses should have. It has been previously noted that service users' and carers' perceptions of their needs and of the help they would like to receive often differ from professionals' views (Barker 1994; Shepherd *et al.* 1995; Murray 1997). Participants in our first study were generally critical of the care they had received from mental health nurses. A 'good' nurse was frequently described by users as someone with the lay qualities of 'common sense', 'warmth and sensitivity', 'being nice' and 'someone who can be a friend'. These findings were consistent with other research which suggests that service users appear to value professionals' interpersonal and 'human' qualities rather than specific therapeutic approaches (McIntyre *et al.* 1989; Ballard & McDowall 1990; Arnold *et al.* 1992; Rogers *et al.* 1993; Lothian Health Council 1996).

What was startling for us was that many participants questioned the role played by nurse education in promoting the qualities they valued. 'Education' was perceived as instilling professional qualities and knowledge in students (as is the

---

[1] Since the time of writing, the UKCC has become the Nursing and Midwifery Council (NMC) and the NBS has become part of NHS Education for Scotland (NES).

Table 6.1   Differences between the 'traditional' approach and a 'user- and carer-informed' approach.

'Traditional' approach	'User- and carer-informed' approach
• Nursing knowledge mainly borrowed and adapted from other disciplines	• Emphasising and valuing users', carers', students' and lecturers' personal knowledge and experiences
• Professionals/disciplines as experts	• Service users, carers and professionals as experts
• Expertise equated with traditional and scientific knowledge	• Expertise equated with personal qualities, knowledge, experiences and resources
• Emphasis on teaching theories about mental health and distress drawn from traditional academic disciplines	• Emphasis on teaching qualities and attitudes. Mental health and distress understood from a personal experiential perspective
• Clear boundaries between professionals', service users' and carers' experiences	• Blurred boundaries between professionals', service users' and carers' experiences
• Objective, problem-focused and promoting 'cook book' nursing	• Subjective, individual-experience focused and uncertain
• Maintaining the status quo of practice and service provision by responding to service agendas	• Challenging and aspiring to change practice and service provision by highlighting users' and carers' agendas

intent). These professional qualities were generally not valued by participants in our study, and indeed could be viewed as detrimental to nurses' ability to help. Participants' perception of professional qualities was linked to their experience of treatment dominated by the medical model of mental illness, which is focused on diagnosis, symptomatology and medication. In our experience this was the dominant model operating in most local mental health services at this time.

Many participants suggested that nurses who had been educated and professionalised through the hospital-based mental health 'system' ended up perceiving and interacting with users as 'text book cases', rather than as individuals with unique experiences of distress. Professional qualities were also seen as eroding the human qualities they valued and this in turn led to 'distance'. Several other authors have pointed out that the use of professional terminology and routine, standardised approaches to care are often the outcomes of professional education and serve as mechanisms for maintaining professional control by distancing (Brandon 1991; Wilkie 1999; Wood & Wilson-Barnett 1999). The view that professional education was in some way detrimental to nurses' human and caring qualities was strongly held by several participants in our study. As one person stated:

The most important thing nurses can do is abandon their training.

We were uncomfortable hearing these views, which obviously conflicted with many of the values then underpinning our curriculum.

Our findings suggested that the conflict between human and professional qualities was of crucial importance. Perhaps the most helpful way to view this is not in terms of a dichotomy, but rather as a continuum with 'human' qualities at one end and 'professional' qualities at the other. Human qualities refer to a nurse's ability to be a 'friend' to users by acting in a sociable and human way. Professional qualities relate to 'professional' knowledge and skills that result from a formal education. Nurses are able to possess both human and professional qualities concurrently. However, the key appeared to be that if a nurse cannot function at the 'human' end of the continuum, progress towards professional help cannot happen. It seemed also that service users, in particular, perceived that nurses needed to find the right balance, be able to recognise the person's needs at any one time, and slide up and down the 'human'–'professional' continuum accordingly. Our findings reflected the need for mental health nurses to progress to a new type of caring, described by Barker and Whitehill (1997) as 'caring with' rather than 'caring for' people. 'Caring with' people implies a partnership, shared responsibility in the caring process and an equal relationship. 'Caring with' may have its starting point in nurses' human qualities and nurses' abilities to focus on and understand the human experience of distress.

Our findings strongly suggested that being able to function as a friendly human being was seen by service users and carers as key, and accordingly that the curriculum should aspire to promote and protect these qualities in students. It seemed that emphasis had to be placed on learning with and from service users and carers, not just learning about professional stereotypes of mental distress. Our findings further suggested that promoting human caring qualities may entail nurses being in touch with their own mental health and periods of distress. It is notable that many users described good mental health nurses as people who 'had life experience', 'had experienced problems themselves' and 'were in touch with their own personal vulnerability'.

The impact of 'the process of involvement' on professional and personal outcomes

An outcome of the first project was a realisation that, while we had consulted users and carers about our curriculum, we had not actually involved them. This realisation drove the second phase of our work. The outcome of the second phase was a strategy for user and carer involvement in the curriculum which has several aims, including the integration of involvement as a major curricular theme (see Risk *et al.* 2000). However, we have persistently observed the importance of the involvement *process* for us, not just the outcomes of it. This was a uniquely *personal* process for those involved and it may be that the impact of our involvement work resulted in personal rather than institutional changes to both conceptualising and teaching mental health nursing. Discussion here draws not only on findings from the evaluation of the strategy development process, but also on a facilitated group reflection undertaken by all lecturers involved in the project, and from personal reflective accounts written by one carer, one service user and two lecturers.

Accounts of how to *do* involvement (e.g. Goss & Miller 1995; English National Board 1996) imply that by following certain key principles, a rational process of involvement can be undertaken. The English National Board (1996) suggested that for user involvement to be a positive and active process it must be underlined by the key principles of consultation, negotiation, partnership and mutual respect.

Little attention has been paid in involvement literature to the *experience* of involvement and the *meaning* of the involvement process for individuals going through it. An overwhelming theme for us was the powerful personal and emotional effects of participation in the second project, illustrated in the following quotations:

> This project has given me back my health of mind, a purpose and direction for that part of my life that I never thought possible. (service user participant)

> My overall experience of being involved is one of the best things that has happened in my time as a carer, to be able to have worked with lecturers and students and other users/carers is one that I would not have liked to miss. It has been a great privilege to have been involved and I look forward to future involvement in the project. The project has made my life as a carer more worthwhile. (carer participant)

The importance of this perhaps indirect yet very positive aspect of bringing all the parties together with a shared aim should not be underestimated. The lecturers involved in the process saw the change in power relationships and identity as a crucial consequence of this process. For example:

> I have learnt a lot and significantly changed my philosophy and feel my involvement has changed my teaching dramatically. I also feel that we have achieved collaborative working and this is probably the most 'equal' my relationship with service users has been in my career. (lecturer participant)

Another powerful element of the involvement process for the lecturers involved was a perceived blurring of roles and identity. While lecturers were ultimately responsible to the funding body for ensuring the project outcomes were met within tight time scales, we eventually retained little control of the project's progress. A decision had been taken by service user, carer and student members of the Project Management Group that lecturers should form only a minority in the sub-groups, minimising our control over the strategy and evaluation. Despite the lecturers' intended 'democratic' approach to the conduct of the study, other group members perceived lecturers as holding ultimate organizational power and consequently as able to disempower other groups involved. Paradoxically, the lecturers experienced their ultimate responsibility and accountability to the funding body as reducing their power, and that reduction as both anxiety provoking and marginalising. Linked to this was a realisation that the boxes we started the project in – 'service user', carer', 'lecturer' and 'student' – represented a false division. In the reflective process following the projects, members of the lecturer group noted that they also had direct experience of mental distress and of acting as carers for family members.

An interesting question to pose is whether lecturers' experience of the involvement process in some way changed us as people and practitioners, or 'rehabilitated' us as mental health nurses towards embracing a different approach to mental health nursing education? Of similar interest is the question that still perplexes us: 'What did the users and carers involved really bring to this process of our change?' We had set the people we worked with the task of curriculum design, a task that daunts even experienced educationalists. The users and carers involved with us had an understandable lack of expertise in curriculum design and delivery and of nurse education. They did not design our curriculum, but instead indirectly shaped and informed it. They shared with us their personal stories of being service users and/or carers and their experience of contact with mental health professionals and services. They also brought naiveté (in a positive sense), a willingness to learn and humility towards higher education that made us see the privileged position we occupy, and the power that is often unconscious and taken for granted. Through this they made us explain and thereby question some taken-for-granted aspects of our knowledge and practice. Ultimately, perhaps the most important things that they brought, and we all shared, were friendship, camaraderie, humanity, kindness, personal support and a willingness to listen to everyone's views as equals, to break down barriers and to learn from each other. In writing this we have been struck by how closely these qualities match those identified in the initial research project where we sought the qualities that users and carers most valued in mental health nurses. This has ultimately taken us towards a version of mental health nursing focused on valuing humanness and using 'experience' and valuing experience as its starting point; a version in which attitudes are as important as (if not more important than) particular skills and theoretical knowledge.

A user- and carer-informed curriculum – opportunities and contradictions

Our journey through the involvement process resulted in our aspiring to deliver a pre-registration mental health nursing programme that promotes human caring qualities in students through emphasising learning with and from service users and carers, not just learning about professional stereotypes of mental distress. Consequently, we have moved towards a curriculum that accords value to, and places emphasis on, service users' and carers' experiential knowledge. However, this does not mean a total rejection of the traditional knowledge bases we previously drew on, nor that we are able to ignore the other stakeholders who drive the pre-registration nursing education agenda.

Our involvement work was a powerful process that inspired and engaged those who took part, and there is no doubt that the greatest changes have been in individual lecturers' approaches and attitudes. However, several changes have also been translated into the curriculum and into the classroom. Within our programme there have been a range of 'curriculum changes' that reflect both an 'embedded' approach and more discrete or 'outcomes'-orientated changes and innovations. The embedded approach is exemplified by the adoption of user and carer involvement as one of the three key underpinning curricular themes for our revised (2001) mental health nursing pre-registration programme. Emphasis is placed on valuing personal knowledge and experience, and at the outset of the programme teaching and learning about mental distress and mental health nursing are initiated by people's stories about experiencing distress and receiving treatment. Alongside teaching and learning about professionally defined helping approaches, students are also exposed to user- and carer-led approaches and literature. Evidence explored on the programme emphasises that user/survivor and carer literature is valid 'evidence'.

Attempts are made to blur the boundaries between professionals', services users' and carers' experiences. The curriculum is underpinned by a philosophy that mental distress affects us all and that it is acceptable for students and lecturers to acknowledge and share their own experiences of distress and caring for people with distress. Emphasis is also placed on the subjective experiences of distress and the underpinning approach to exploring distress is through the eyes of those experiencing it. This has resulted in a move away from teaching from a 'diagnosis, signs and symptoms and nursing care of' approach to approaches that are more individually-focused and uncertain. Other discrete outcomes include the regular formal monitoring of programmes and modules by users and carers to ensure that the user and carer perspective is given equal attention alongside professional perspectives. Modules have been developed that focus explicitly on implications of involvement for practice, and on anti-discriminatory practice. Components of students' practice assessments now include user and carer feedback to students whilst on practice placements.

Although the former English National Board (1996) made it clear that user and carer involvement should be 'more than slotting people into the curriculum', the educational literature to date has taken a somewhat narrow or 'classroom'-centred view of the potential impact of user and carer involvement on education. This view could be seen as tokenistic or as 'passive involvement'. Whilst it was an overriding concern that we wanted to go beyond 'just wheeling in users and carers to tell stories', there has been a marked increase in the number of sessions involving or delivered by users and carers.

We have bought into an approach that primarily reflects the interests of users and carers and accords at least equal weight to people's experiential knowledge compared to traditional academic knowledge. Our discussion thus far has focused on how the processes and outcomes of involvement work have informed our approach to teaching mental health nursing. It is important to note that various contexts structure the forces that condition mental health nursing education and mental health nurses' work. Our approach to teaching mental health nursing has to operate in the context of different forces pulling in different directions regarding knowledge and we also have to attend to the various other interest groups that try to shape the field of mental health nursing to their own advantage. Recognising that aligning ourselves with a particular stance produces various conflicts, tensions and discrepancies, we will now reflect on this by considering our stance in relation to our own institution and wider institutional contexts.

We are acutely aware that the impact of our involvement work has resulted in personal changes in the way lecturers conceptualise and teach mental health nursing, rather than any institutional changes within Napier. A major theme to emerge from the process evaluation of the strategy development project, relating to the experience of being involved with the project, was the constant high levels of energy and commitment that were needed to drive forward the project and the emerging approach to the curriculum. There were (and still are) particular concerns among the lecturers involved about whether this momentum is sustainable over a long period, particularly without the support of the wider university. There were pressures on lecturers to train and support project members – who had little or no experience in the tasks of strategy development and evaluation nor of working within the pressured environment of current higher education practices – whilst grappling with learning 'involvement' themselves. A key part of the strategy was the identification of institutional structures needed to support a user- and carer-informed curriculum in the long term. Part of this was the need, identified in the 'Strategy for Involvement', to appoint a specialist Project Development Worker. This worker was to have a key role in supporting users and carers involved in the curriculum and keeping the momentum of involvement alive. It is pertinent to note that despite concerted efforts to achieve external and/or internal funding for this post, this has not been achieved.[2] The drive to continue to develop and maintain a user- and carer-led curriculum comes mainly from the lecturers involved in the original project, rather than reflecting an institutional policy.

Other areas of tension are also obvious. While we have related an approach to mental health nursing education in this chapter, it may be that this is a personal approach constructed by the authors and not one embraced by all lecturers in our team. Just as the *process* seemed to be crucial in 'involvement', *not* being part of the process was perhaps central in others feeling excluded. The involvement projects appear not to have been wholly embraced by *all* the lecturers in the team. With few exceptions the membership of the project team remained unchanged for the duration of the project. Lecturers not involved with the project expressed some feelings of being excluded and felt that there was '*a risk of a small number of people having promoted this project over a number of years with no fresh blood*'. It is also noted that those not directly involved saw the 'involvement

---

[2] A part-time User and Carer Involvement Development Worker was appointed in September 2003, funded internally by the Faculty of Health and Life Sciences, Napier University.

projects' as rife with political correctness, and those driving the involvement movement as attaining an almost cult-like status. While we have outlined a range of curricular changes as outcomes of the process of involvement, it is notable that most of these have been instigated by the academic team members directly involved in the involvement projects.

The major forces that necessarily shaped our (and others') most recent version of the pre-registration curriculum are the recommendations of the UKCC Commission for Nursing and Midwifery Education outlined in *Fitness for Practice* (UKCC 1999). This creates further tensions in responding to the user and carer agenda and in producing a curriculum that is informed primarily by the experiential knowledge of service users and carers. Despite the fact that the need to involve service users and carers in mental health services, care and education has long pervaded policy, academic and practice accounts intended to shape and drive the future of mental health nursing, this is not mentioned in *Fitness for Practice*. Rather, future trends in health care are perceived as relating primarily to greater demands being placed on nurses' 'technical competence' and 'scientific rationality'. The agenda in *Fitness for Practice* recommendations is service-driven, not consumer-driven, and emphasises the preparation of practitioners fit not only for practice but primarily for employers' purposes. Consequently, across the UK, pre-registration programmes have now been designed and implemented on 'outcomes-based, competency principles', an approach with potential to be bureaucratic, restrictive and reductionist (Girot 1993; Le Var 1996). This approach does not sit comfortably in the context of our programme.

It has been challenging for us to reconcile these two contrasting approaches and philosophies to curriculum development. *Fitness for Practice* suggests an approach primarily about training nurses to meet the needs of the service, and our approach aspires towards training people to respond to the needs of people experiencing and caring for those with mental distress. Difficulty in reconciling the two approaches perhaps also signposts a major omission in our involvement work. Our involvement projects excluded involvement of trained mental health nurses, who provide support and mentorship to students. In retrospect, we think this deliberate decision taken at the outset of the projects might further polarise us and service providers. There are also concerns that our philosophy and approach may set up for our students unrealistic expectations of practice. In the limited evidence to date about the impact of user and carer involvement, Wood and Wilson-Barnett (1999) concluded that students did take a 'more user centred approach to care' as a result of user involvement in the classroom. These outcomes of involvement could also be seen as adding yet more fuel to the 'theory–practice gap' by encouraging students to adopt a critical stance on practice and perhaps instilling unrealistic expectations among students that they can challenge and change practice. Further research needs to address whether the knowledge and attitudes that the students have gained through this process lead to changes in practice settings towards a more 'user-centred approach', or instead lead to a further decline in standards of care as a result of students leaving a 'system' that they see as unwilling or unable to accommodate the philosophy of 'involvement'.

Another potential limitation of our having shaped our curriculum via involvement work is that we have bought into an approach that primarily values users' and carers' experiential knowledge and we have used this to shape a particular version of mental health nursing. However, the knowledge base we drew on was largely based on consulting and eventually working with a relatively small, and perhaps *unrepresentative*, group of users and carers. There are two aspects to the 'representativeness' debate in involvement work of this nature. The first is to do with whether the group recruited for the project represented a methodologically sound research sample. In this case we acknowledge potential criticisms regarding the 'representativeness' of the users and carers we consulted. The number of people we involved was small and we did not give a voice to all relevant and interested parties. It is also worth noting other limitations of our work in relation to the second aspect of 'representativeness', namely whether we consulted and involved a sufficiently wide range of participants to ensure representation of breadth and diversity of experience. Maybe we made the mistake of considering mental health service users as a homogenous group with similar experiences and views. This mistake perhaps also reflects professional and patronising attitudes towards mental health service users as undifferentiated rather then unique individuals. It became clear as the involvement progressed that, of course, different people hold different views. People consulted during the first project who were recruited from users' forums tended to be much more critical of mental health services and nurses, and proposed an active role in curriculum design and delivery. People who attended 'drop in' centres tended to be slightly less critical of services and did not appear to desire an active role in the curriculum. The suggestion was made (by service users attending 'drop in' centres) that consultation and involvement should be left to the 'experts', the 'experts' being user forum members and activists. One could argue that this reflects a perception among users that user activists are empowered to represent other users' views. Therefore we acknowledge the risk that the people we have worked with could become the 'unelected representatives' of all mental health service users and carers. Beresford (1994) points out that one of the concerns most often raised by service providers is the 'representativeness', and consequently the legitimate expertise, of service users and carers as knowledge informers. This is a contentious issue and many people in user organisations feel that service providers challenge their representativeness in order to invalidate what the users say, or exclude them. Beresford points out that a double standard may be at play here with the representativeness of policy makers and professionals rarely challenged in the same way.

It is also essential to ponder the notion of expertise. Our approach assumes that all service users and carers hold unique and expert experiential knowledge. Rolfe (1999) makes an interesting point (in relation to practitioners) that experience and expertise should not necessarily be viewed as interchangeable terms. Rolfe argues that 'expertise' and 'expert status' can only be accorded when clinical experience has been internalised and used wisely for the benefits of others. Perhaps it is this distinction between *experience* and *expertise* that needs to be explored in the debate around user 'representativeness' and 'representation'. Users' own experiences will only be seen as valid 'evidence' when internalised and used to inform the experience of others in the wider user/carer community. We consider that this constitutes true representation and expertise. Otherwise users are seen merely as individuals armed only with their own experiences and hence 'unrepresentative' and lacking 'expertise' in the experience of other users.

Mental health nursing now also operates within the prominent context of the evidence-based health care agenda. This agenda values 'scientific' knowledge as the true form of 'expertise'. Within this agenda the valued 'gold standard' knowledge is based on findings from quantitative research, particularly randomised controlled trials. This poses an additional conflict regarding how user-generated and carer-generated experiential knowledge is valued within mental heath nursing education and practice. Although 'expert opinion' is increasingly seen as an important (and overlooked) aspect of 'evidence' in the context of evidence-based health care, 'expert opinion' is usually construed as practitioners' opinions (with a passing mention of patient preference). Thereby a practitioner's clinical experience and expertise confers expert status (McKenna 2000). The literature of evidence-based health care not only fails to ascribe this status to user/carer experience or expertise but indeed seeks to 'de-emphasise intuition and unsystematic clinical experience' (Evidence Based Medicine Working Group 1992), to which status user and carer experience might be relegated. Thus, user and carer accounts of individual experience might be seen as directly opposed to evidence-based health care as currently constructed.

References

Arnold, C., Finucane, J. & Rose, N. (1992) *The First 24 Hours*. Manchester: MIND.

Ballard, C.G. & McDowall, A.W.T. (1990) Audit in practice – psychiatric in-patient audit: the patients' perspective. *Psychiatric Bulletin*, 14: 674–5.

Barker, P. (1994) Points of view. *Nursing Times*, 90 (8): 66–8.

Barker, P. & Whitehill, I. (1997) The craft of care: towards collaborative caring in mental health nursing. In: *The Mental Health Nurse: Views of Practice and Education* (ed. S. Tilley). Oxford: Blackwell Science.

Beresford, P. (1994) *Changing the Culture: Involving Service Users in Social Work Education*. London: Central Council for Education and Training in Social Work.

Brandon, D. (1991) *Innovation Without Change: Consumer Power in Psychiatric Services*. London: Macmillan.

English National Board (1996) *Learning from Each Other*. London: ENB.

Evidence Based Medicine Working Group (1992) Evidence-based medicine: a new approach to teaching the practice of medicine. *JAMA*, 286 (17): 2420–5.

Forrest, S., Brown, N., Risk, I. & Masters, H. (1998) *User and Carer Involvement in Curriculum Design and Delivery*. Report prepared for the National Board for Nursing, Midwifery and Health Visiting. Edinburgh: Napier University.

Forrest, S., Risk, I., Masters, H. & Brown, N. (2000) Mental health service user involvement in education: exploring the issues. *Journal of Psychiatric and Mental Health Nursing*, 7: 51–7.

Girot, E.A. (1993) Assessment of competence in clinical practice: a review of the literature. *Nurse Education Today*, 13: 83–90.

Goss, S. & Miller, C. (1995) *From Margin to Mainstream: Developing User and Carer Centred Community Care*. York: Joseph Rowntree Foundation.

Le Var, R. (1996) NVQs in nursing and midwifery: a question of assessment and learning? *Nurse Education Today*, 16: 85–93.

Lothian Health Council (1996) *What makes good mental health services?* Report of the Consultation with People Using Mental Health Services in East Lothian and Midlothian. Edinburgh: Lothian Health Council.

Masters, H., Forrest, S., Harley, A., Hunter, M., Brown, N. & Risk, I. (2002) Involving mental health service users and carers in curriculum development: moving beyond classroom involvement. *Journal of Psychiatric and Mental Health Nursing*, 9: 309–316.

McIntyre, K., Farrell, M. & David, A. (1989) Inpatient psychiatric care: the patient's view. *British Journal of Medical Psychology*, 62 (3): 249–55.

McKenna, H. (2000) Evidence-based practice: demolishing some myths. *Nursing Standard*, 14 (16): 39–42.

Murray, I. (1997) How can clients and carers become allies? *Nursing Times*, 93 (27): 40–42.

Risk, I., Masters, H., Forrest, S. & Brown, N. (2000) *Involving service users and carers in curriculum design and delivery: a strategy for involvement*. Report prepared for the National Board for Nursing, Midwifery and Health Visiting. Edinburgh: Napier University.

Rogers, A., Pilgrim, C. & Lacey, R. (1993) *Experiencing Psychiatry: Users' Views of Services*. London: Macmillan/MIND.

Rolfe, G. (1999) Insufficient evidence: the problem of evidence-based nursing. *Nurse Education Today*, 19: 433–52.

Shepherd, G., Murray, A. & Muijen, M. (1995) Perspectives on schizophrenia: a survey of user, family, carer and professional views regarding effective health care. *Journal of Mental Health*, 4: 403–422.

United Kingdom Central Council for Nursing, Midwifery and Health Visiting (1999) *Fitness for Practice – The UKCC Commission for Nursing and Midwifery Education*. London: UKCC.

Wilkie, P. (1999) Commentary: signs of action on the long path to user involvement. *NT Research*, 4 (4): 271.

Wood, J. & Wilson-Barnett, J. (1999) The influence of user involvement on the learning of mental health nursing students. *NT Research*, 4 (4): 257–70.

Chapter 7

Involving Individuals in Mental Health Nursing Education

Mary Chambers, David Glenister, Carol Kelly and Tessa Parkes

This chapter is dedicated to the memory of Pete Shaughnessy, a committed survivor activist and co-founder of Mad Pride who fearlessly taught others. His work continues through those he inspired.

Introduction

Ensuring the access of users and former users of mental health services to mental health nurse education might, if successful, enrich the experiences of other staff and students and ultimately users and carers. The specific contribution of this chapter is to examine the involvement of individuals in mental health nursing education, and specifically the involvement of users and former users. There is already a large literature on the role of institutions in learning and we believe it is time to redress this balance through a consideration of the role of individuals.

The task for the authors of this chapter was to write together about the role of experiential knowledge of mental health crises in the curriculum of mental health professionals, in particular mental health nurses. We outline some of our thoughts about experiential knowledge as a different way of knowing that cannot merely be placed alongside other ways of understanding mental distress/illness. However, experiential knowledge is commonly viewed as at best peripheral rather than core in the understanding of, and education about, mental distress or illness. We highlight the strange relationship between this very personal human knowledge and the impersonal curriculum most mental health students are exposed to (where the emphasis is almost exclusively on the treatment of symptoms, with the vital separation of 'them' from 'us') the treated from the treaters. We end the chapter by investigating the transformative potential of experiential knowledge and the possibility of a re-evaluation of the role of experiential knowing in the future curriculum of mental health nurses.

Before doing this, we need to put our writing in context. This chapter is a collaborative venture between four people who are committed to user involvement in mental health nursing education but who come from different positions and vantage points. Some of us have personal experience of mental health crises and some of us do not. Some of us have responsibility for the curriculum content of mental health nursing courses and some of us do not. This obviously affects what we have to say and how we communicate that. This shared chapter has consequently not been easy to write. As authors attempting to write together through several drafts over a considerable time period we have sometimes strengthened the boundaries between ourselves, rather than transcended them.

Writing, sharing and learning

This chapter is a place where we as co-writers have struggled with the task of articulating the role of experiential knowledge in nursing education. We have been faced with examining our own ways of writing and working with others in the light of this task. This personal work continues, but we hope some of what we write about here may connect with others who are attempting what we have decided to call 'shared learning across difference'. We have used the practice of reflexivity to help us articulate these difficulties – both to each other and to readers.

Reflexivity, according to Freshwater and Rolfe (2001: 529), has different meanings to different writers. In their view two main interpretations are predominant: reflexivity as the process of turning thought or reflection back on itself, and reflexivity as the process of turning action or practice back on itself. In this chapter we use reflexivity to mean both reflection on thought *and* practice or behaviour, as our shared writing has naturally involved both thinking together and working together. Reflexivity is a tool that can be used to demand that we look closely at form as well as content, process as well as product. It forces us to make links between our actions and our intentions, our inner selves and the outer selves we present to others. As co-writers we used reflexivity and conversations to communicate our common ideas and then integrate our distinctive voices and allow ourselves the opportunity to really hear what each was saying. We also use reflexivity as a communicative device throughout this chapter.

One particular dynamic of our shared writing was a reliance on a technological means of communicating our ideas about shared learning (email), rather than talking to each other face-to-face and exploring issues as people together. We discovered that trying to share learning about experiential knowledge in this way worked to squeeze out the important communication dimension that takes place when people get together to work out ideas and core values. Technological communication such as email can be fast and incredibly useful in many co-writing exercises, but in this case it impeded us massively. This was because we failed to really communicate as individual people, and hence wrote our pieces very much in isolation; not engaging openly and deeply with what each was contributing. In other words, we related through 'head talk', rather than as whole people relating and acknowledging our personal experiences, values and beliefs.

Crucially, this approach to shared writing and shared learning did not work because it did not allow us to articulate properly what we were trying to write about – experiential knowledge of mental health crises and the centrality of this to the curriculum of mental health professionals. Experiential knowledge is, by its nature, intrinsically personal and individual. Experiential knowledge is not like other forms of knowledge more commonly peddled in mental health education. It is radically different. It emerges from our personal and individual interpretation/understanding of extreme states of mind and body, and our own personal and individual human reactions to such extreme states. Knowing about human distress and the extremes of human experience, because one has experienced them, is therefore a different kind of knowing than that gained by reading research and theoretical ideas about mental illness produced by mental health professionals, social and/or biological scientists. This kind of knowing cannot be merely additional to other ways of understanding mental distress/illness; rather, it should make us look at all other knowledge anew. We shall return to this idea later in the chapter. Thinking of experiential knowledge as just another kind of knowledge that could be written about as one would write about other kinds of knowledge was an early mistake we made in writing this chapter.

Our early, rather mechanistic approach to shared writing did not enable us to create something with an energy or synthesis of its own: a shared product. For that to work we required an approach that could not only link four different individuals' ideas together in a logical fashion that would make sense to readers, but also link us as individuals; an approach capable of articulating both the distinctiveness of our voices and the commonalities. We think that many exercises involving survivors and users in the curriculum work in ways similar to our early efforts, and produce isolated and mechanistic interventions that are not long-lasting or meaningful. In the case of our shared writing this was due to lack of time and lack of attention to opening up honest and regular dialogue. It was also due to a preoccupation with creating content, and consequent neglect of process, something our later reflexive work together challenged. Again there may be similarities between this and the involvement of survivors and users in the mental health curriculum. Finally, it also seemed to characterise our general reluctance to attempt to integrate 'academic' and more personal writing styles or narratives. Bringing these two very different styles of writing and knowing together was profoundly challenging, as we will illustrate.

A return to lecturing

The following was offered by one of the authors, describing his experience of returning to work after an extended mental health crisis.

Teaching without knowing
The classroom is full of noise. Laughter. Gossip. A smell of youthful exuberance and perfumed soap. I bang a desk and a reluctant silence falls. I am not the man I was. No longer so assured and arrogant. No longer obese or experiencing the sour mouth taste of last night's alcohol. Still tall.

Who are these women? Working class wives seeking something more than home, children and husband. Single mothers seeking to escape poverty and isolation. Young women rather wilted from dancing last night away, looking to revive themselves as soon as the student union bar opens. An occasional studious look. Each with their own life story. Their own triumphs, and their own tragedies. I know little of them.

Who am I here? You know, the one who was sick. Told us all about it last year. Unspeakable terror, he said. Moved by unseen forces, he said. The emergency domiciliary visit from the psychiatrist. Thought she was an impostor, and didn't answer her questions. Threw the medication down the toilet. Thought it was poison. Strangely enough, resulted in tinnitus ever since. Was drinking too much too. Never been the same since. What are we doing here? They see me, but I don't see them. There is so much information to be given out. DSM-IV diagnostic classification. Aetiology. Treatments. Slip in a little on unorthodox understanding and responses. They look keen to learn. Many notes are taken. Acetates are shown. The words are well-rounded and sentences securely structured. A voice filled with the awfulness of mental illness, and at the same time hope for the future. Anxiety adds a certain edge of urgency, and plea for understanding. So much information to impart, perhaps so little learnt. How much learning is lost in teaching? If we were to know each other, even attempt to understand each other, how much teaching would then be necessary?

I cannot read like I used to. He thought the birds were speaking to him singing of long lost tales. Exemplar of psychosis. He thought his life was wasted, and thought through methods of suicide in great detail. Exemplar of severe depression. I still read of this but I can no longer accept these clinically composed snapshots, spare me the dull and dry cookbook of cognitive recipes for a better life.

Let me take you all to the wild woods, where the wild things roam. Let us write large words together with a long staff on the sandy solid track through the pine tree wood. Let us pan for the gold of wisdom, you and I in the river of life. Sometimes I will look after you. Sometimes you will look after me. Sometimes we will go our separate ways. Let me come to love my madness and you to love yours. Let us not live in fear of awesome majesty of the mind. I tread without knowing, my words like fish in the river, but hoping that something of the value of my experience of madness shines through.

The author offered this to the other authors, without further explanation. For him, at that time, there was little more to be said. However, the other authors were bewildered, uncertain how to use the writing. Here was experiential knowledge, but where did it fit in a book chapter about experiential knowledge? The result was silence and mutual incomprehension, for several months, between all authors. Later, the author himself wrote that he was attempting to convey a tender transparency of self, a greater consideration of others, resistance to medicalising and psychologising discourses, and the necessity of learning through madness. As the author shifted to exploring his experience, to explain it to others, communication commenced again. The irony was that in an academic book about forms of knowledge, an offering of raw experiential knowledge initially appeared a problem to accommodate. Later, from this experiential knowledge was to emerge the main theme of this chapter: the individual within the institution.

Individualisation

The lack of a facilitative environment in infancy and childhood, suggests Winnicott (1965), can result in loss of opportunities for the development of integration, interdependence, integrity and identity. Mental health crisis can be understood in positive terms as an attempt to address these losses. If this understanding is to occur, a facilitative environment is needed to offer opportunities previously not available for the development of integration, interdependence, integrity and identity which were previously not available. Regrettably, such an understanding of crisis as an opportunity for maturation is rare in mental health services, and as a result opportunities for individualisation are lost.

To some extent, mental health education shoulders some of the responsibility for this limited understanding. Mental health practitioners can hardly be expected to *create* facilitative environments if they have not experienced them. The opportunities for integration, interdependence or indeed integrity within mental health education are surprisingly limited. The focus upon a range of competencies can militate against the serious consideration of character, which too easily is reduced to appraisal of popularity among staff and students. If the supposed accomplishments of professionalism are adopted without an inner personal maturation, the result can be a mask of limited value to users, carers or the practitioners themselves. In short, the parallels between the maturation of the service user and the maturation of the student mental health practitioner, and their respective experiences of facilitative environments, must be thought through and intrinsically connected with the curriculum.

The extent to which this can be undertaken depends upon the level to which those individuals who lead the design and delivery of the curriculum themselves have a healthy sense of integration, interdependence, integrity and identity. All too often this maturation is assumed. The possibility that individuals who have thought through these issues at depth for themselves, as a result of mental health crisis, are well placed to offer leadership should be seriously considered. It seems to us, therefore, that individuals who have used mental health services and alternatives to mental health services should play a central role in the design of the curriculum because of their knowledge of individual maturation.

Teaching 'us and them'

In mental health practice education, standard scientific knowing is exemplified in the observation of signs and the elicitation of symptoms, and the consequent formulation of a diagnosis. This necessitates a social distance between the scientist and his or her objects, the knower and the known. Subjective emotive reflections upon sensations, thoughts, feelings and intuitions are discounted unless they assist with diagnosis. Students soon learn this.

One of us remembers an incident very early on in her nursing training. When one of the patients asked where she lived, she told the person. She was then reprimanded by a senior nurse who told her that one of the golden rules of being a psychiatric nurse was to not give out personal information. The rationale was that giving out personal information would place nurses at risk from patients. The underlying reason was that becoming professional involved becoming less personal, even to the extent of becoming less of an individual person. This felt very uncomfortable for the student nurse, who had previously not seen her interactions and relationships with individuals in this way. Just to add to the confusion, around the same time the student nurse was told about an incident another student had witnessed, on a different ward in the hospital, in which an elderly man had been badly beaten with his walking stick by one of the male nurses. While nurses can sometimes be at risk from patients, it is equally true that patients can be at risk from nurses (Glenister 1997; Williams & Keating 1999). However, anecdotes such as these are not uncommon as examples of ways in which it is the patients who are constructed as 'different' and 'dangerous'.

Related to this, and central to the reason why experiential knowledge of mental distress is so marginalised, is the belief that people who have experienced mental health problems are not as able, as bright, as resilient and as competent at life as people who have not experienced mental health problems. In research on user involvement undertaken by one of the authors (Parkes 2002), a service user observed:

> The view of the person who's mentally ill is that we're thick, we're not very bright and we're lifelong, that is that we're going to have this diagnosis forever. We aren't ever going to work again, we probably won't have kids, if we did, it wouldn't be wise. That's the common attitude of a lot of staff that I've come across, that you're not normal, that you're a severe case of schizophrenia or whatever. The majority seem to see us like that, we are not encouraged to get a job or have a life or have an input even in services.

Mental health service users are viewed as rather faulty and overly needy human beings who will have 'lifelong' problems of living. This attitude is palpable throughout most mental health services, in our view, and is a major reason why user knowledge and knowledges have thus far largely been ignored; a 'don't encourage them' approach. Service users describe this attitude toward them on the part of individual professionals, and on the part of whole services more generally, as massively disempowering and confidence-destroying. Indeed, this is one of the main complaints about mental health services from users and survivors (Chamberlin 1988; Deegan 1990, O'Hagan 1993; Rogers *et al.* 1993). Such attitudes prevail despite many challenges from enlightened workers, intellectuals and user activists. This may be due in part to the continued teaching of 'us and them' in mental health education that also still prevails.

Living without barriers

Another of us offered two pieces of writing that described her experience of living with mental health problems/crises. The first is a poem; the second, part of a narrative.

Waiting in the lobby of the hospital
Waiting in the lobby of the hospital,
All my friends have left me,
Even Steve and Sal.
Only left to my emotions,
Which they tell me, lie to me.
They tell or they suggest that I am not normal, and yet I feel normal.
Oh no – just a little confused – a little bemused at what is going on.
Doctors, nurses, staff seem to wait behind, out of sight but not out of mind.
They seem to wait for my next reaction,
For my next attraction to another human communication.
Communication, that is what is lacking, that is what they are attacking.
Even with all my courage, I cannot eat, I cannot speak, and even left beside me
The brown–grey liquid, called 'Hot Chocolate', is not touched.
Everyone is so nice here, the staff that is.
All my other comrades seem to laugh at me.
All the shades of black humour which surround this condition,
This omission of reality.
For the cold, hard world outside, that once opened the door to me,
Has seen me lying on the floor, stripped naked of my self-respect,
The blatant image that reality was too hard, and too coarse for my finer feelings.
That is what it was like, yes, that is what it was like.
So now I find a brave world, good but fair,
Where kindness and caring are not just part of someone else's working day,
Measured out to each lost cause, to help them on their way.
No, it's not like that anymore,
Now when I try at something, it is not a false praise that I get,
Though praise is less than it once was, it is at least meaningful.
Not dressed up in uniform like an army dame.
The world is kinder to me now.
And the reality which I have, is not questioned at every turn,
Is not something which I have to learn.
The person which I find each day is me –
A somewhat shy, somewhat quiet thinker,
In a non-thinking world.

That is why I wrote this, for you to think,
For you to think, 'Thank God I have my sanity'.

At this time my ambition was

At this time my ambition was to be a millionaire so I took up a degree programme in Estate Management where only 5% of the students were female. After we were divided into groups I was the only female in my group. Within six weeks I had become reclusive, isolated in the halls of residence and speaking to no one. On being summoned to the Welfare Officer's department I imagined that I was in a siege situation. Terrified I found myself in a psychiatric hospital for six weeks without any visitors or any form of personal support. I was unable to talk or communicate and was diagnosed as a catatonic schizophrenic.

On returning home for Christmas I was admitted to a local psychiatric hospital where I had a lengthy stay. The following year, 1978, I was allowed back to university but as I was heavily drugged with prescribed medication I kept falling asleep during lectures. This went unnoticed and I failed four of my six examinations. On receiving my results I was taken to the Welfare Officer again where her assistant berated and humiliated me for failing my exams. The lecturers responsible for the course advised me to take a law degree, as that was the only examination in which I had obtained a high grade.

Deflated and humiliated I returned home and worked locally as a lifeguard. For the following eighteen months I undertook a course in sports studies at a local university. During the first year I was highly popular, being the year representative for my course. Despite being on medication and consequently overweight I passed both the physical and the academic components of the course achieving marks close to the top of the group.

In the summer of 1981 my illness manifested itself again, this time as bipolar depression. During this summer I had two jobs; one as a student industrial cleaner, the other as a swimming and volleyball instructor. Once when out with friends they encouraged me to stop taking my medication, which I did. On one occasion after this I went on a drinking binge in the city. I ended up in the police station, something which I did frequently during the course of my illness. I would call into the police station and chat up the officers and then leave. However, when I was particularly ill on one occasion the police called my uncle to take me home. During this bout of illness I engaged in other behaviours such as going around pretending to be a child psychologist. On another occasion I visited a friend's house and put Stelazine in the Rice Crispies.

As my behaviour deteriorated I was admitted to a psychiatric hospital where I spent six months. Part of my time in hospital was spent in the locked ward. Throughout my stay in hospital I was reassured by the medical profession that I would be able to resume my studies as soon as I recovered. Around this time I had been selected to play volleyball at a national level. Unfortunately a major tournament had to be cancelled due to rioting so my opportunity to play was limited as no facilities existed in the hospital. Indeed the hospital administration abolished the position of recreation officer so there was no organised sport in this large hospital. The lack of exercise and the medication caused me to gain four stone in weight. When I finally presented myself back at the college I did not resemble an athlete.

At this time the director of studies, the psychologist and the medical doctor considered me unfit to resume my studies despite my having passed all of my exams. They told my mother who came with me that medically I was not fit as I could suddenly develop mania on a mountain or in the swimming pool and be a danger to others and myself. No other course would take me into second year and I could not get a grant to repeat a first year in another subject. I therefore spent eight years in the wilderness saving to get the money to go university. In the meantime I discovered I could pursue my athletic career as a swimming and life saving instructor.

I had spent four years battling against the prescribed drugs and the authorities, both medical and educational. They had all made false promises and put up barriers. Finally at the age of 30 I was able to go through university and eventually passed my Masters degree in Peace Studies. This happened because of regular counselling and support on a friendly campus and the long-suffering love of my late mother.

Again, different points can be taken from this personal narrative in terms of the things that hindered and supported this author's educational experience. The lack of support and understanding by university personnel could be highlighted as a contributing factor. Or the role of gender and isolation could be emphasised in causing the stress or distress in the first place. A different reading of this text could highlight the struggle against medical and academic humiliations and false promises, and ultimate success as a peacemaker. The author, in another piece of writing, places emphasis on the importance of support, counselling and love from family members as some of the most crucial factors in helping her succeed in an educational environment. She reflects:

> Had there been a system in operation whereby people like myself could have received counselling and a befriending system and more support throughout the first year, then I may well have passed without impairment.

Having personal pieces of writing such as these offered to the chapter meant it was impossible to produce a straightforward, ideas-based chapter together, however much this was the approach we had started with and some of us had initially preferred or assumed we should take. In the same way that user knowledge in its diverse forms challenges the validity and status of other previously taken-for-granted knowledge, these pieces of personal writing challenged the other authors to consider their positions, actions and approach more carefully. These pieces meant that we had to start communicating more openly and honestly if we were to be able to co-create something of value. They forced the issue. As stated above, experiential knowledge can be transformative in this sense because it forces us to re-evaluate what we know and how we know what we know.

Transforming knowledge

Integrating knowledge about the human experience of crisis, loss, mental distress, mental illness – however we wish to describe it – into the curriculum of health and social care professionals will necessarily be fraught with difficulty. This is so in part because of the investment thus far in approaches to the study of human distress that have marginalised such knowledge and continue to do so; more importantly because those who do not have personal access to such knowledge often undermine the status of this knowledge because they do not understand it, perhaps even fear it.

Opening up the professional curriculum to experiential knowledge about human experiences that can be described as madness or mental illness exposes the rest of the curriculum to scrutiny in new ways in: profoundly challenging ways. Bringing this knowledge and understanding truly into focus risks the rest seeming irrelevant if not totally misguided. It takes a lot of commitment and energy to really see the wood *and* the trees: to really ask 'What does this new knowledge mean for me and my previous understandings/misunderstandings?'.

Experiential knowledge, if acknowledged at all, is largely seen as peripheral rather than core to the understanding of mental distress and illness. However, incorporating user knowledge in its diverse forms into the curriculum meaning-fully cannot be done without the rest of the knowledge changing too – by virtue of the fact that much of it no longer makes any sense whatsoever in the light of this new knowledge. We cannot continue with our prescriptive, individualistic, interventionist recipes for 'mental health' in the face of knowledge that demands a different frame of reference. Knowledge about the extremes of human experi-ence cannot be 'tacked on' to existing structures, especially ones that have con-tributed to the diminution of the status of such knowledge.

Institutions

When examining the relationship between universities and mental health services it is prudent to look back at the origins of these institutions. There is a strange association between universities and mental health and learning disability services, and this results in a lack of recognition of their reciprocal roles. Doerner's (1982) history of class and madness provides an opportunity to examine the nature of their relationship. In contrast to the declining aristocracy and its exemplification of tradition the emerging industrial bourgeoisie sought to exemplify reason, to themselves and to others. The mental health services of the day, the asylums and the learning disability colonies respectively, were pioneered by the emerging bourgeoisie as monuments to their mastery of madness (Doerner 1982). The detail of difference was that while asylums (mental health services) were for those deemed to have lost reason, the colonies (learning disability services) were for those deemed never to have found reason. The development of the modern university, accommodating the new industries such as engineering, was, in contrast, an edifice of reason. Asylums and colonies, and universities, were insti-tutional exemplars of the separation of the unreason of madness and reason.

The university and the mental health service remain today almost mirror im-ages of each other. The university seeks to assist individuals to conquer the high peaks of reason, while the mental health service seeks to rescue individuals from the depths of unreason. The university student sharpens the steel of his or her intellect, the mental health service user drowns in the depths of unthinkable sorrow, or ecstasy, or is caught in traps and snares of faulty thinking. The former are deemed capable of conquering social heights, the latter deemed in dire need of care and control, preferably out of sight from others. Any individual who wishes to travail both peaks and depths will be treading a lonely path.

The juxtaposition, or positioning side-by-side, of the university and mental health services shakes this institutionalised societal separation of unreason and reason. This was less problematic when it involved the relatively small numbers of medical and clinical psychology students, but is more problematic now that it involves much larger numbers of nursing and social work students. Students experience this as a gap between the university and health services, between theory and practice, and between themselves as students in the university, students on placement and individuals with family and friends. There is, in the juxtaposition, the possibility of a profound psychological integration of thinking and feeling, deep insights afforded by both intellect and intuition, and the soaring of the mind grounded in the sensation of the body. However, this is precisely what has not happened. The integration of either institutions or individuals would require a fundamental shift towards the acknowledgement and accommodation of the individualisation of users, students and indeed staff alike, social planning towards individual and institutional maturation and, furthermore, an avoidance of discrimination.

User/survivor experiences of employment and education

The belief that people who have experienced mental health problems are 'faulty and needy' and the stigma associated with this has obvious real consequences beyond the bounds of mental health services. The experiences of people when they try to get back into work or into education are now well documented (Perkins *et al.* 1997; Rooke-Matthews & Lindow 1998; O'Flynn & Craig 2001; Bertram 2002). Rooke-Matthews and Lindow's (1998) research, for example, showed that many people working in mental health services, both in the voluntary and statutory sector, reported discrimination by employers, colleagues and educators. For an individual to be open about being a current or former user of mental health services, whilst in employment or in education, requires bravery and stamina. As Pearson (2001) has described, because mental health problems are often invisible, the onus is on the individual to disclose that he/she has a history of using services, rather than this being self-evident, as it may be for people with some physical disabilities. So people often choose not to disclose this information because of the dangers associated with being honest about this aspect of one's life.

People who have used mental health services frequently encounter prejudice and stigma in the workplace. They experience patronising attitudes and ignorance and may face active attempts to make them leave their jobs. In research on user participation within mental health services (Parkes 2002), people who identified themselves as user-workers described having 'invisible pats on the head' from colleagues or managers when they succeeded in doing something well; expectations of their performance were so much lower than for their co-workers. There were also examples of user-workers being carefully observed by fellow professionals, and of normal behaviours (such as frustration and sarcasm) being interpreted as the person becoming unwell. For one user-worker, speaking out in a meeting against Trust cuts resulted in her GP increasing her medication and threats of being sectioned and admitted to hospital (Parkes 2002).

Discrimination is reported not just in employment settings; it has also been reported in professional mental health education and in in-service training. In Rooke-Matthews and Lindow's (1998) research, students who had used mental health services described mental health professional educational environments as discriminatory. Some of the reasons for the difficulties experienced were: being sent on placement where they had been service users; being presented with an image of mental distress which emphasises the medical aspects, implies low expectations of service users and lowers their self-esteem; being faced with forms of mental health prejudice from staff and students which they felt they could not confront directly; and fearing that their service use would be discovered if they went through a difficult patch or were using mental health services while a student.

So, for many people, disclosure is not a risk worth taking. This means that the number of people with experience of mental health issues or of using services, who are working in mental health services or studying to become mental health professionals is largely unknown. This reinforces the invisibility of users and former users as mental health professionals, educators and students, which in turn makes it harder to give full attention and recognition to the role they can play in addressing the issues raised above; namely personalising and individual-ising the curriculum through experiential knowledge. So what needs to take place for their place and position to be recognised and fully integrated?

The involvement of users and survivors in the curriculum

Survivor and user involvement in mental health education has become a standard requirement for the General Social Care Council, formerly the Central Council for Education and Training in Social Work, and the English National Board for Nursing, Midwifery and Health Visiting. However, how far this has been imple-mented and with what success remains difficult to judge. Bringing survivors and users in to provide isolated one-off input, rather than attempting to involve people more meaningfully, is still common. This can be tokenistic in the same way that many attempts to involve survivors and users in the delivery and planning of mental health services have been (Croft & Beresford 1992; Barnes & Bowl 2001; Parkes 2002). Attempts to negotiate all or substantial parts of the curriculum with survivors and users are rare (Masters *et al.* 2002). Comparisons can be drawn between this and the initial demands for increased student involvement in educa-tional curricula. It could be argued that student involvement in higher education curricula has become very much a marginal activity in otherwise-unchanged institutional structures, with student representatives sitting on the odd committee or board meeting with little real power or credibility.

'Institutionalised resistance' to innovations in survivor and user involvement in the mental health curriculum, similar to that found in service provision settings (Parkes 2002), is likely to be encountered if there is a serious attempt to move beyond these tokenistic efforts. Repper *et al.* (2001) offer graphic descriptions of the experience of users involved in the development of a curriculum for a nursing degree programme. Professional language was used, which led to users feeling alienated, and survivors/users were asked to endorse statements rather than generate ideas (Repper *et al.* 2001). Repper *et al.* (2001) concluded that the involvement of survivors and users was more of a token gesture than a real desire to have them shape the curriculum.

Becoming loud and proud – the transformative potential of experiential knowledge

Because of the extent of discrimination faced by people who have experienced mental health crises and distress, both in mental health services and in wider society, it becomes necessary to look to models of practice that challenge such discrimination, in order to move forward. Antidiscriminatory practice, as described by Thompson (2001), can provide one way of uncovering and then challenging and combating discrimination. The promotion of equality in mental health nursing education settings involves breaking down some of the barriers we have explored in this chapter. It would involve acknowledging the current discriminatory practices that are largely ignored or denied by educators. It would involve encouraging people with experiences of mental health crises to enter the mental health professions as students, professionals and educators, and their peers valuing the experiential knowledge and understandings that they can bring.

We also believe that experiential knowing itself can be a vehicle for changing the deeply ingrained cultures and attitudes that persist in mental health services and educational settings. The mere presence of university staff and students who have used mental health services can shake some of the deeply held assumptions within mental health education. This is because their presence can undermine the comfortable contrast between the recipients of care, survivors and users, and those who educate mental health practitioners. The aspiration is that such shaking results in a more creative mental health education, fostering not only professional but also personal growth.

Giving experiential knowledge a central place in the mental health nursing curriculum would also disrupt fundamentally the way that nurses have traditionally been taught to prioritise the recognition of symptoms over an individual's experience and interpretation of these experiences and their meaning. It would destabilise the 'us and them' culture. Experiential knowledge has the capacity to be transformative, not merely additional to other ways of understanding mental distress/illness, because it makes us revisit the other things we think we know with new vigour. Experiential knowledge forces the issue and asks us to truly evaluate the validity of different knowledges and ways of knowing. However, the integration of users' and former users' experiences in curriculum design and delivery would necessitate a willingness to listen and learn from highly emotive and rich descriptions.

While agreeing with Freshwater and Rolfe's (2001) argument for transformative learning through reflexivity, we contrast their advocacy of learning among professional peers with our attempt to learn across difference by bringing together individuals with professional and/or personal knowledge of distress and mental illness. Our own transformative learning would probably not have occurred if only professional peers had written together. It only occurred through tolerating discomfort and the diversity of forms of knowledge with a view to learning from each other. Rather than placing transformational learning through reflexivity within a project of professionalisation, we are seeking to socialise transformational learning through reflexivity, in pursuit of individual, institutional and also societal change.

We began this chapter by asserting the need to refocus on the role of the individual rather than the institution in mental health nursing education: the role of the individual user, individual student, individual professional and individual educator. We have argued that emergence of stronger individuals may be accomplished through a planned maturational environment in both practice and educational settings. If the process of individualisation was pursued with the same vigour as the process of institutionalisation is at present in mental health practice and education settings, the outcome of mental health education might then be radically different: individual practitioners of the future fully alive to themselves and others, sensitive, subtle and skilful.

Strong individuals are to be found among users, who have often pursued personal and social change with courage and commitment despite enormous adversity. These individuals are also sometimes strong enough to work with their own weaknesses. Such individuals have much to offer in curriculum design and delivery. There is also a need for strong individual educators who acknowledge and accommodate the diversity of forms of knowledge, and different ways of knowing, in themselves and others, especially when this is difficult and even seemingly disruptive, and yet still are positive and purposeful in their work. Such individuals also have much to offer in curriculum design and delivery. Strong individuals who can transform their own and others' learning through social reflexivity, and who share a hatred of old injustices and a commitment to making a just peace, may in time transform their own communities.

References

Barnes, M. & Bowl, R. (2001) *Taking Over the Asylum: Empowerment and Mental Health*. New York: Palgrave.

Bertram, M. (2002) Vocation and inclusion: what are the issues? Proceedings of the Association of Occupational Therapists in Mental Health, 6th Annual Conference, Abstracts. *Mental Health OT Special Issue*, 7 (2): 26.

Chamberlin, J. (1988) *On Our Own*. London: MIND.

Croft, S. & Beresford, P. (1992) The politics of participation. *Critical Social Policy*, 35 (12): 21–45.

Deegan, P.E. (1990) Spirit breaking: when the helping professions hurt. *The Humanistic Psychologist*, 18 (3): 301–313.

Doerner, K. (1982) *Madmen and the Bourgeoisie: A Social History of Insanity and Psychiatry*. Oxford: Blackwell.

Freshwater, D. & Rolfe, G. (2001) Critical reflexivity: A politically and ethically engaged research method for nursing. *NT Research*, 6 (1): 526–37.

Glenister, D. (1997) Coercion, control and mental health nursing. In: *The Mental Health Nurse: Views of Practice and Education* (ed. S. Tilley). Oxford: Blackwell Science.

Masters, H., Forrest, S., Harley, A., Hunter, M., Brown, N. & Risk, I. (2002) Involving mental health service users and carers in curriculum development: moving beyond 'classroom' involvement. *Journal of Psychiatric and Mental Health Nursing*, 9: 309–316.

O'Flynn, D. & Craig, T. (2001) Which way to work? Occupations, vocations and opportunities for mental health service users. *Journal of Mental Health*, 10 (1): 1–4.

O'Hagan, M. (1993) *Stopovers On My Way Home From Mars: A Journey into the Psychiatric Survivor Movement in the USA, Britain and the Netherlands*. London: Survivors Speak Out.

Parkes, T. (2002) *Feathers and thorns: the politics of user participation in mental health services*. PhD thesis. Canterbury: University of Kent at Canterbury.

Pearson, A. (2001) *Progress through partnerships*. Keynote Address at the Massey University Disability in Education 35th Annual Conference, September 2001, Albany, New Zealand.

Perkins, R., Buckfield, R. & Choy, D. (1997) Access to employment: a supported employment project to enable mental health service users to obtain jobs within mental health teams. *Journal of Mental Health*, 6: 307–318.

Repper, J., Felton, A., Hanson, B., Stickley, T. & Shaw, T. (2001) One small step towards equality. *Mental Health Today*, December: 24–27.

Rogers, A., Pilgrim, D. & Lacey, R. (1993) *Experiencing Psychiatry: User Views of Services*. Basingstoke: Macmillan Press/MIND.

Rooke-Matthews, S. & Lindow, V. (1998) *A Survivor's Guide to Working in Mental Health Services*. London: JRF/MIND.

Thompson, N. (2001) *Anti-discriminatory Practice*, 2nd edn. Basingstoke: Palgrave.

Williams, J. & Keating, F. (1999) The abuse of adults in mental health settings. In: *Institutional Abuse Across the Life Course* (eds N. Stanley, J. Manthorpe & B. Penhale). London: Routledge.

Winnicott, D.W. (1965) *The Maturational Processes and the Facilitating Environment: Studies in the Theory of Emotional Development*. London: Hogarth Press and the Institute of Psychoanalysis.

Chapter 8

Models of Mental Health Nursing Education: Findings from a Case Study

Ian Norman

Introduction

This chapter draws on findings of a research study carried out for the English National Board for Nursing, Midwifery and Health Visiting (ENB) between 1993 and 1995, which aimed to identify the changing educational needs of mental health and learning disability nurses in the light of community care reforms (Norman *et al.* 1996) and two papers published subsequently[1] (Norman 1998a, b). During this study the research team was struck by respondents' divergent views about the nature of these nursing specialities and the implications of these views for nurse education. We noted, in particular, the debate between those who advocated a specialist educational preparation for either mental health or learning disability nurses and those who favoured generic preparation of nurses from all specialities. The generic–specialist debate was relevant to nursing as a whole at the time of the study, but was a major concern to mental health nurses, many of whom felt that the trend towards generic education threatened what they perceived as the distinctive nature of mental health nursing.

The chapter outlines models of nurse education discerned through analysis of data from the ENB study, and interrogates them to draw out their central features and assumptions about mental health nursing as a practice discipline. In conclusion the chapter comments on the current relevance of these models to mental health nursing in the UK. The emphasis is on mental health, rather than learning disability nursing, reflecting the focus of this book; but the models are relevant to both specialities, both of which are less well rooted in the biomedical tradition than general nursing.

Background

The role and educational preparation of mental health nurses has been under scrutiny since the closure of the old psychiatric hospitals, in a way that did not

---

[1] Permission has been given by the publishers.

arise when most nursing was hospital-based. As Nolan and Hopper (2000) point out, the strength of the old hospitals lay in their structure. This structure did not encourage mental health nursing to develop and flourish, but it did provide nurses with a sense of security. Mental health nurses' roles, their remit and responsibilities and the value base of their discipline are less clear today than in the past, and fewer nurses feel that sense of security experienced by their predecessors.

Divergent views on the roles and priorities of mental health nurses were reflected in the varied perceptions of desirable pre-registration education programmes for mental health nurses, gathered for the ENB-funded study referred to above. Topical questions at the time of the study included: should students be prepared much as before with an allegiance to a single professional status? Or should a variety of options be available to prepare nurses to work flexibly in different settings and specialities? Team working across professional and organisational boundaries is widely regarded as essential for high quality care (DoH 2000b) and so questions arose about how to best prepare nurses who are most likely to contribute to effective teamwork. At the same time there are new demands on, and priorities for, mental health services. One such is the unequivocal priority of people with severe and enduring illness, which requires service providers and education commissioners to make sound and discriminating judgements about the level and type of educational preparation of nurses to meet local requirements.

The specialist–generic debate in mental health nurse education

Within the discipline of mental health nursing in the UK the specialist–generic debate has a long history. Indeed, many educational developments can be viewed as attempts by mental health nurses to distance themselves from general nursing. The 1952 General Nursing Council (GNC) psychiatric syllabus reflected the view that mental health nursing was very similar to general nursing. Anatomy and physiology featured strongly, psychiatric topics not being covered until the final year. In 1957 an experimental syllabus was introduced based on the concept of 'situation-centred teaching' which emphasised that subjects taught, which now included psychology and psychiatry in the first year, should be applicable to direct patient care. This approach to teaching was endorsed in the 1964 GNC psychiatric nursing syllabus which comprised three areas of study: the human individual; concepts of mental disorder; and skills needed to deal with mental disorder – preparation of patients for procedures and investigations, administering drugs and monitoring their effects. A substantial amount of the syllabus continued to focus on human biology, psychophysical disturbance, physical illness and first aid.

However, the view that mental health and general nursing were similar was questioned to an extent by a major review of psychiatric nursing in 1968 by the then Ministry of Health. Amongst other recommendations the report identified the need for psychiatric nurses to develop skills in psychotherapy. This view resonated with views of opinion leaders of the time such as Altschul, who had endorsed interpersonal skill development several years previously (Altschul 1964). Ten years later Harries (1978) pointed out that many nurses had developed such skills experientially mainly in those services that had evolved as therapeutic communities.

The 1974 psychiatric nursing syllabus continued along the same lines as the 1964 syllabus, but for the first time introduced sociological concepts and teaching on community care and gave more attention to services such as occupational, recreational and industrial therapy. It also advocated increased specialised teaching from doctors, social workers and other therapy professionals.

During the 1980s, which were characterised by cutbacks in NHS spending and changes in the law concerning people with mental health problems, a new emphasis was placed on nurse training. The Judge Report on nurse education stated the need to better educate and widen the knowledge base of nurses by improving links between schools of nursing and hospitals (Royal College of Nursing 1985). The report highlighted the need for students to be treated as learners and not used as a cheap labour force, and argued for teaching both concepts and practice of care. It did not, though, specify how this balance should be achieved nor how to support newly trained nurses in practice, how to teach nurses basic management skills, how to avoid duplication of effort between professions and how to cope with inter-professional rivalry.

Although those involved in the education debate were looking at ways of meeting community needs and raising nurses' morale, nursing academics and the Psychiatric Nurses' Association became concerned about what they perceived as a move towards the generic practitioner (Mangan 1992; Thomas 1993). What followed was a revised nursing syllabus for psychiatric nurse education in England and Wales (English National Board for Nursing, Midwifery and Health Visiting 1982), which appeared at a time when the view that institutional psychiatric care was a thing of the past and community care its natural replacement went unchallenged (Weller 1989). The 1982 psychiatric nursing syllabus emphasised nursing skills and had a very different emphasis than the 1974 syllabus; the latter having been essentially a list of content to be covered during the course. According to Thomas (1992) the skills emphasis was prompted by a desire of the authors to define the skills of the psychiatric nurse, highlight self-awareness as a prerequisite of all therapeutic interventions, and stamp psychiatric nursing as a 'human activity'. We see the influence here of Peplau's concept of psychiatric nursing as a therapeutic and interpersonal process in which the nurse and patient are active partners in a mutual learning experience (Peplau 1952). Although Peplau had been a major influence on psychiatric nursing in the USA through publication of her *Interpersonal Relations in Nursing* in 1952, further writings and her contribution to graduate psychiatric nurse education at Columbia and Rutgers Universities, her ideas were to enter UK psychiatric nurse education only slowly, and it was the late 1970s and early 1980s before they became prominent.

A major theme of educational developments up until the mid-1980s was to highlight the distinctive contribution of psychiatric nursing, and to distance it from general nursing. However, it was not long before separate moves were to completely undermine this initiative and reunite these branches of nursing under the single banner of Project 2000 (UKCC 1986). Project 2000, the government's major reform of nurse education in the 1980s, aimed to reverse the steady decline in nurse recruitment by raising the status of nursing. In doing so, Project 2000 emphasised the common ground between different areas of nursing, in particular mental health and general nursing care. As a result, all students on the Project 2000 course had to take the Common Foundation Programme (CFP) spanning the first 18 months.

The Royal College of Nursing (1993) pointed out that, as far back as 1968, the Joint Sub-Committee of the Standing Mental Health and Standing Nursing Advisory Committee had acknowledged the important relationship between psychiatric nurse training and the quality of mental health nursing (Ministry of Health 1968). That committee had concluded that separate training and qualification (registered mental nurse) was essential. Some 35 years later this same issue remains prominent in the debate on nursing education. In 1962 psychiatric nurses were required to take the same intermediate examinations as general nurses, with specialisation following thereafter. It seems to many somewhat ironic that the Diploma in Higher Education – Nursing (DipHE) format for the 1990s would require mental health and learning disability nurses to do much the same.

Project 2000/DipHE was the result both of an extensive consultation process and of a costing exercise by the auditors, Price Waterhouse. Their favourable financial report did much to convince the government of its benefits (Jones & Jones 1992). By creating specialists trained to at least diploma level, who would be sufficiently flexible and resourceful to cope with most circumstances, the DipHE course would produce skilled professionals ideally suited to meet the challenges of community care at minimum cost. Thus, the community reforms provided an opportunity to maximise the use of a then-decreasing supply of resources, in what was perceived to be the most efficient and cost effective way, while also – in many cases – avoiding the need for expensive retraining to fit hospital nurses for work in the community (Jones & Jones 1992).

In summary, it is difficult to piece together the many influences on mental health nurse education from the 1950s to the beginning of the new millennium. However, at the time that the ENB commissioned the study reported here, Project 2000 had been running for more than five years and there was growing concern about its impact on the minority branches. Although Project 2000 had been designed to raise standards and morale, some writers (e.g. White *et al.* 1993) had begun to criticise the greater emphasis in the CFP on general nursing at the expense of the specialities (in particular mental health and learning disability nursing). In addition, there were growing doubts about the clinical credibility of nurse lecturers within the new university departments and their ability to deliver an education relevant to the rapidly changing needs of a community-based mental health service. Further, there was lack of clarity about the educational needs of mental health nurses following implementation of the NHS and Community Care Act (1990).

The study

The purpose of the study was to identify the changing educational needs of nurses involved in the practice of mental health and learning disability nursing in different settings and to make recommendations to the ENB concerning educational programmes for these nurses. Our aim was to highlight emerging issues that demanded the attention of educators.

Research design and methods

The purpose of the study led us to engage in two kinds of activity: discovery of existing progressive practice in care provision of mental health and learning disability services – a task for systematic inquiry; and development of models of educational provision that might guide policy makers, educationists and practitioners in the future. These two activities of discovery and development followed three phases: preliminary work, fieldwork, and analysis and model development. The research design took an 'embedded multiple-case study' approach as described by Yin (1989). That is to say, the study consisted of two 'cases', one in mental health and one in learning disability service provision. The 'multiple data points' within each case were represented by the respondents in three sites – three in mental health and three in learning disabilities. The proposition investigated was that the educational needs of mental health and learning disability nurses are influenced by changing practices in service provision towards a more community-based service. The purpose was to gain a broad view of the issues under investigation rather than to compare non-representative sites with each other. Use of multiple sites provided the mechanism for collecting views from a diverse sample of respondents within each case. Thereafter the data were aggregated across sites within mental health and learning disability and across both specialities.

Phase 1: Preliminaries

Three activities comprised Phase 1.

Key informant interviews: Interviews in the form of guided conversations with 22 key informants helped us identify research sites and substantive issues for inclusion in interviews with respondents in these sites. The key informants for each nursing speciality were selected along the lines of a snowballing approach. It was not our intention to select a representative sample; rather, it was to locate people from diverse disciplines and occupations who had strong views on the subject of our inquiry. This strategy ensured that the sites selected and the content of the interview schedules reflected the range of issues important to service provision and education in mental health and learning disability care.

Selection of sites: Six sites in England were selected using the following criteria:

- Type of service (three in mental health and three in learning disability)
- Stage of development (in transition or fully operational)
- Service provision (progressive, i.e. perceived to have made attempts to address the issues under the Act)
- Educational links (collaborative).

We sought a diversity of care provision, context and educational links in a purposively selected sample of cases. Three mental health sites were located, one each in London, the northwest and the south of England. The learning disability sites were in London (a different area from the mental health sites), the northwest of England (same area) and the Midlands.

Developing interview schedules: Interview guides were developed and tested for relevance and feasibility in the first study site. No single interview guide would have been suitable for all respondents, hence six were developed for: service managers and 'workers' (nurses and support workers involved in direct care); college lecturers; service-users and carers; advocates; student nurses; and other stakeholders (e.g. other health care professionals, executive managers and purchasers).

The guide for service managers and workers was the longest and covered the following areas:

- The organisational structure of the service
- Locating the respondent in the organisation
- The process of user referral and management
- Principal components of work
- Educational experience and its contribution to role performance
- The nature of the respondent's work in relation to other health professionals
- Aspects of service delivery related to the Act
- The respondent's vision for service development and its educational implications over the next five years.

Phase 2: Fieldwork

The fieldwork took place between November 1993 and October 1994. A total of 147 people were interviewed, 88 in mental health and 59 in learning disability services.

Phase 3: Analysis and model development

Responses to each question were analysed across all six interview schedules; for mental health and learning disability respondents separately, and for the total sample. The responses were classified into 'views' that summarised a topic area and these were grouped into 20 categories and seven themes, which are reported elsewhere (Norman 1998b). The final stage of analysis sought to draw on the data to build normative, or ideal, models of mental health and learning disability nurse education. Those models relevant to mental health nursing are the focus of the rest of this chapter.

The models

An important theme that emerged from a large number of respondents was that nurses in both specialities were seeking a role distinct from, but collaborative with, other professions. Several respondents reminded us that the identity of mental health nursing in the past had been linked closely with hospital care and with psychiatrists. In an attempt to free itself from what was perceived to be medical domination, mental health nursing was developing its own ways of working; some beneficial, such as forging closer bonds and alliances with users, but others less so, such as the trend towards isolationism. A key informant cited as evidence of this isolationist trend the nursing models movement and mental health nursing textbooks of the 1970s, which deliberately eschewed psychiatric terminology in favour of an obscure American–English nursing jargon.

Samson (1995), in a paper published around the time that we were writing the project report, argued that medical dominance in British psychiatry may be fracturing as a result of the policy switch towards community mental health services and the managerial reorganisation of the health services. Several respondents reported that doctors have lost considerable influence to social workers and clinical psychologists, and so supported Samson's view. Some respondents felt that mental health nurses were also in danger of losing influence because of their medical links, and that they needed to re-establish their identity. In this regard they welcomed the emphasis of the review of mental health nursing, undertaken during the course of our study (Department of Health 1994), on nurses establishing a partnership with users. This emphasis was welcomed by many respondents as providing nurses with a distinct focus of activity and a unique identity within the mental health care professions.

A minority view was that mental health and learning disability nursing should be combined. An opinion leader who was one of our key respondents pointed out that the separation of mental health and learning disability nursing is an historical accident. Combining them again would reflect the organisation of psychiatry, which covers the full range of psychiatric problems. Moreover, the interventions needed by these two client groups are broadly similar. Both groups need information, support and help with how to cope. The target of intervention with learning disability and mental health clients is the mind; mental health clients have limited reasoning and learning disability clients have limited understanding (so the leader's argument went). Thus the mind is the root of their problems. This is not so much the case for people with physical illness (even though

Table 8.1 Summary of the ideal models of mental health nurse education.

	Specialist	Pragmatic	Unity of nursing	Generic
Desirable pre-registration training structure	• Distinct from general nursing • Direct entry MH/LD – diploma level	• Distinct from general nursing • DipHE offers best chance to retain distinctiveness • Clear role definition needed	• Nothing distinctive about specialities – as general nursing • DipHE allows practice of common skills with different patient groups	• Single (probably graduate) nursing qualification • Specialist post-registration
Nurses' knowledge	• Therapeutic relationship basis of direct care • Humanistic psychology • Social sciences • Experiential learning	• As 'specialist' • Dedicated curriculum time for speciality • Teachers qualified in and value the speciality	• Common ground across nursing specialities • Psycho-social nursing • Flexible teachers across branch programmes	• Common ground across nursing specialities • Biomedicine • Management studies • Supervision of non-registered workers
Expectations service users	• Person-to-person relationship	• As 'specialist' + • Good care environment/packages • Distinct nursing contribution within multidisciplinary teams	• Patients have common needs which all nurses should be able to meet	• Relationship not always necessary • Planned care package • Medication management
Shared learning? Joint training?	• Yes some – mainly at post-registration level • No joint training	• Yes some – mainly at post-registration level • No joint training	• Yes – across the family of nursing • Moving towards single nursing qualification	• Yes – across all nursing specialities • Probably – common core across health care disciplines
Advantages	• Attractive to willing and able care workers • Wide entry gate	• DipHE offers best chance to stem rising tide of genericism	• Rising tide of genericism welcomed	• Raised status of academic nursing • High-calibre recruits • Flexible, proactive workforce

it may have psychological effects) whose care is properly the province of general nurses.

A counter-argument, which was put forward by other key informants, points out that the 'combined' model makes a false and simplistic distinction between mind and body. Also, in reality, the needs of the two user groups are very different; one group is ill, the other is not. Moreover, the objectives of care are not the same. With a fair proportion of mentally ill people at least, recovery can be expected and with some conditions (e.g. affective disorders) a cure. By contrast, the objective for clients with learning disability is to lead as normal a life as possible in the community; recovery and care relate to disease and illness, and so are not appropriate. So there is a conceptual difference between the two groups although both do have specific educational needs that are rather different from those of patients with physical illness.

On a similar tack a key respondent with a mental health nursing background supported the idea of learning disability nursing being a post-registration qualification for mental health nurses. The argument presented is that with genetic screening there are essentially two kinds of learning disability client: those with brain damage who need physical nursing, rehabilitation nursing and mental health nursing; and those who need help to lead as independent a life as possible. This second group is the province of social workers, although nurses may be helpful for people with profound and challenging behaviour problems. The great majority of learning disability respondents did not consider that their discipline is best linked with mental health nursing. For them the important debate was whether it was best placed in the 'family of nursing' at all, or allied to social work.

There was widespread agreement amongst our respondents that mental health nursing needed to establish itself at the forefront of community-based services, but there was disagreement as to how this might be achieved, in particular whether pre-registration education should follow a specialist or generic route. This debate is relevant to nursing as a whole but was intensified in the context of our study because genericism was perceived by many of our respondents as a threat to the minority branches – especially to those branches (arguably mental health and learning disability) that are not rooted in the biomedical tradition of general nursing. The debate was perceived by many respondents as central to the future of the two nursing specialities and we drew upon the strong views expressed to develop models of future educational preparation.

The models are expressed as ideals that represent reality, but do not necessarily reflect it. They are presented here as caricatures of the views that emerged, so their distinguishing features are clear. Thus the models are heuristically designed to bring together diverse ideas and stimulate debate.

The models are summarised in Table 8.1. Two are clearly independent: the specialist and the generic models. The other two – the pragmatic model and the unity-of-nursing model – draw upon the first two to support the Diploma in Higher Education (Nursing) programme which was, and continues to be, the dominant form of pre-registration nurse preparation in the UK. One other model

– the social care model – was developed by the ENB study team, but this applied to learning disability nursing only and so is not covered here.

Each model is examined, taking into account the following points to bring out its characteristics:

- The desirable structure of pre-registration nurse education and academic progression in mental health and learning disability nursing
- The basis of nurses' knowledge and the emphasis of the pre-registration curriculum
- The perceived expectations of service users
- Attitudes to shared learning and joint training
- Perceived advantages and disadvantages.

Model 1: The specialist model

The essence of the specialist model is direct entry to single-qualification pre-registration courses in mental health nursing.

Desirable structure of pre-registration training and academic progression

Specialists mourn the passing of dedicated specialist courses leading to registration in mental health nursing, that occurred as a result of the DipHE reforms. Most specialists advocate their revival but as courses based in higher education linked to academic qualifications. Most also support pre-registration courses at diploma level and resist a wholesale move to an all-graduate profession. To make this move would, they argue, effectively exclude from the profession, simply on academic grounds, many people who have the potential to form helpful relationships with people who are mentally ill. In any case, abandoning diploma-level training would simply mean that NHS Trusts will recruit more vocationally trained care assistants and that opportunities for direct personal contact and the develop-ment of therapeutic relationships between qualified nurses and people with mental health problems will decrease.

Opportunities for post-registration education should enable diplomate mental health nurses to build upon an academic qualification while progressing in their professional careers. Courses are available, but many specialists emphasise the importance of building on therapeutic skills, particularly those in the humanistic psychology tradition (e.g. counselling and psychotherapy courses).

The basis of nurses' knowledge and emphasis of the pre-registration curriculum

The reason for specialist preparation is the distinction between mental health nursing knowledge and skills on the one hand, and those of general nursing on the other. The specialist mental health nurse builds a therapeutic relationship between nurse and user as a vehicle for planning interventions in partnership with users and carers. Delivery of care is directed at helping users cope with the problems in living associated with their illness and make progress towards mental health.

This direct personal relationship is crucial to mental health nursing. It is a constant in the user's life and the heart of mental health nursing under all systems of service delivery (e.g. case/care management, team nursing, primary nursing). For some mental health specialists the exercise of the nurse's therapeutic relationship is most vividly expressed in his or her capacity to stick with and maintain relationships with long-term seriously ill people who experience recurrent health crises and periodically exhibit disturbed and aggressive behaviour. Nurses' capacity to defuse and deal with aggressive situations is another hallmark of high-quality mental health nursing which, by virtue of their training and much face-to-face contact with users, they do better than other mental health care professionals.

Specialists recognise the importance of having a grasp of biomedical aspects relevant to mental health care. However, the emphasis for most is primarily on the social science base of nursing practice, in particular communication theory and developing interpersonal therapeutic skills that draw particularly upon humanistic psychology, counselling and psychodynamic psychotherapy. Popular teaching methods include role-play and other forms of experiential learning and an emphasis on supervision in clinical practice.

Expectations of service users

Users value their personal relationships with mental health nurses and first and foremost they want nurses who have the personal qualities and skills to forge such relationships. Mental health and learning disability nursing education should therefore draw primarily on the social sciences and interpersonal psychology rather than be based in the largely biomedical tradition of general nursing. Specialists argue that if qualified nurses withdraw from their direct care role, users will increasingly distance themselves from biomedically-based services; parts of North America were cited where this has already occurred.

Shared learning and joint training

Joint training with other health and social care professions leading to dual qualifications is rejected by specialists because it clouds the distinctiveness of the nurse's role and fudges the issue of what different occupational groups do and should be doing. Moreover, there would have to be good reason for having two occupational groups with overlapping roles when there could be one. However, some shared learning is advocated and there are many possibilities for this, particularly in post-registration education. Shared learning in pre-registration education, particularly with social workers, is also favoured because the basis of the curriculum aimed at building, fostering and using interpersonal relationships for both professions is similar. Some shared learning with general nurses is also possible as long as the distinctiveness of mental health nursing is recognised.

Mental health nurses point to strategies for shared training for mental health and also learning disability nurses and social workers in the 1970s as evidence of the pioneering spirit of these specialities. However, some specialists argue that this work had limited impact because it did not fit the plans for general nursing. General nursing is seen as a dominant force exercising undue influence on the direction of the minority branches of DipHE courses. Merging mental health with learning disability nursing has been proposed but so far has received little support from either speciality.

Advantages of specialist education and critique of genericism

Children at school often gain experience of caring for people with learning disability and mental health problems as a component of general or community studies courses and the fact that many find this an attractive job is confirmed by the number of able and energetic people working as unqualified social workers in voluntary organisations and statutory services throughout the country. These people are committed to a psychosocial approach to care and might go so far as to reject any profession associated with the 'medical model'. They are more likely to be attracted to social work, through the NVQ or diploma route, than to nursing. General and mental health nurses are a different breed. Unqualified people currently working in mental health services are not interested in general nursing; the stereotype of general nursing, which is grounded in the medical model, does not appeal to them. They could, though, be attracted to mental health nursing if it was separated from general nursing. As long as general nursing experience remains a major part of pre-registration nursing education as in DipHE courses, these potential entrants will be lost to the profession. Specialist dedicated courses are much more likely to recruit this highly desirable group.

The current DipHE programmes dilute mental health nursing expertise. This is inevitable in a generic programme. General nurses, through sheer weight of numbers and a stronger foothold in higher education, sway the curriculum towards the biomedical tradition and emphasise aspects of that tradition that are seen as most relevant to nursing general patients. A generic preparation (Model 2) will simply exacerbate this problem and is a luxury that mental health nursing cannot afford. Mental health nursing is a psychosocial activity and much biomedical knowledge gained is redundant in practice.

A generic preparation of three years followed by a further period of specialist practice (Model 2) is detrimental to service users because nurses will inevitably be steeped in and unable to throw off the biomedical tradition of general nursing. Moreover, the cost of increasing the length of pre-registration nurse education will simply price nurses out of the health care market without any benefits to service quality.

Model 2: The generic model

Generic preparation can take several forms. One distinction concerns whether generic education extends across a range of health and social care groups, or is confined to nursing. Generic education within nursing can lead to dual nursing qualifications (entry on more than one part of the register) or a single Registered Nurse (RN) first-level qualification for all nurses; this is the form of generic preparation with which the generic model described below is concerned.

Desirable structure of pre-registration training and academic progression

In retrospect, DipHE courses established under Project 2000 are an unsatisfactory halfway house. DipHE was a move towards generic preparation, which was compromised by fear of the expense and repercussions of losing the student labour force to the labour market. Genericists argue that nurse education should have had the courage not to compromise and instead to go for a generic three-year preparation for all nurses, based in higher education and leading to the RN qualification, perhaps modelled on some programmes in North America.

Many genericists favour three-year programmes leading to a first degree in nursing. Indeed, implicit within some notions of genericism is the assumption of an all-graduate nursing profession. Other genericists would accept three-year courses leading to a diploma or a first degree. Following this, students could choose to do a specialist year, or possibly more, in their chosen speciality. They would be clinically based, probably working as a basic-grade staff nurse for the first year of specialised practice, and would progress thereafter.

Post-graduate qualifications would comprise a portfolio of options at different academic levels that would suit people specialising in mental health/learning disability care. These post-graduate courses would be pursued through a combination of practice and study.

The basis of nurses' knowledge and emphasis of the
pre-registration curriculum

The therapeutic relationship, as espoused by specialists, is not a reality in most services. Economic pressures mean that there is a constant push to look for more cost-effective ways of delivering direct care. Thus it is simply not feasible for nurses to protect their direct care role.

Creating good care environments in a range of client care settings and, increasingly, supervising vocationally trained assistants is now a primary role for mental health nurses. Nurses are best placed to do this because they have a strong grounding in the biomedical tradition and also a foot in the social sciences, both of which would feature in a well-planned generic education programme. An all-graduate nursing profession grounded in an initial generic preparation, in which nurses are freed from the role conflict and drudgery of service commitment, will increase the status of nurses within multiprofessional health care teams. This will enhance their professional confidence and enable them to make a more robust contribution to the creation of care environments than hitherto.

There is much overlap between the skills and knowledge of all nurses. Nursing comprises the application of common skills across a range of human need and over a 24-hour, 7 days-a-week period. The emphasis of the pre-registration curriculum differs from that of the specialists. For genericists the key to the future is flexibility and they see the attempt of specialists to protect traditional direct care nursing roles as part of a professional protectionist agenda. If nursing is to flourish within cost-effective services it must adapt to a variety of service delivery patterns. Nurses must have the confidence and ability to leave behind their direct care role with patients and take on a wider brief. Skills of management and leadership are highly valued as the key to nurses managing and developing services to meet users' needs. These skills are linked to newer forms of service delivery, such as case/care management.

The close relationship between mental health/learning disability nursing and general nursing locates all of nursing primarily in the biomedical tradition. Genericists see this as completely appropriate to the new care arrangements for mental health and learning disability users. These nurses recognise themselves as grounded in health and health care and this requires much closer allegiance to the biomedical model than has been the case for many years. Let social models be the province of social workers, they say.

Expectations of service users

Users value their personal relationships with nurses, but relationships with health care assistants can be just as beneficial if these people are properly supervised as part of an integrated health care service. Moreover, not all mental health service users need close relationships with nurses. What is important is careful assessment of the level of support individuals require and providing a planned package of care to address that need.

Specialist preparation of mental health nurses over 35 years has yielded few positive benefits for users. The growth of the user movement has highlighted deficiencies in mental health nurses' knowledge and skills; some nurses' limited interest in and knowledge about long-term medication management of seriously mentally ill people and inadequate knowledge of the physical illnesses experienced by users being two examples. Many of these deficiencies result from mental health nurses' neglect of the biomedical origins of the profession, their tendency to work independently from other members of the health care team and their relatively low status vis-à-vis other health care professionals. A move to generic education can improve the conditions under which nurses currently work.

Shared learning and joint training

Joint training for all nurses at pre-registration level is favoured. Some genericists see this as just the beginning of a transformation of health care disciplines by extending joint training across professional groups and creating new varieties of health care worker. Others are just as cautious as specialists regarding joint training with other disciplines, and on similar grounds; it clouds the distinctiveness of nursing and fudges the issue of what different occupational groups do and should be doing.

Shared learning is favoured by genericists and there are many possibilities for this, in particular in issues raised by service delivery systems on which all workers need information and need to reach agreement (e.g. record keeping, confidentiality, advocacy, principles and procedures of referral).

Advantages of generic preparation and critique of the specialist model

In many ways the DipHE course represents the worst of all possible options for mental health nursing. The dominance of general nursing throughout the curriculum, particularly in the CFP, means that, in effect, generic nurse preparation has arrived already by the back door. The result is a badly thought through pre-registration education for mental health nurses. Moving purposefully to a generic three-year pre-registration programme, so expanding the existing CFP to three years, gives the minority branches much more opportunity to be clearly and fully represented.

Specialists go on about the importance of the therapeutic relationship, but it is not a reality in most services. The result of pre-registration nurse education leading to a single mental health qualification has yielded few positive benefits for users. In seeking to distance themselves from general nursing, specialist mental health nurses have neglected the biomedical tradition to the extent that they have increasingly distanced themselves from doctors and have not exercised the influence that they should on developing progressive health care services.

Specialists are swimming against the tide of unfolding events. Pressures for cost containment and the trend towards the generic nurse in other European countries mean that the UK generic nurse is inevitable. The important thing is to seize the moment and make generic preparation as good as it can possibly be for nurses who elect to follow the minority specialisms.

Nursing, particularly mental health nursing, holds little appeal for well-qualified people who are able to make a difference to the shape and quality of service provision. The trend in cost-efficient services is towards fewer knowledgeable and skilled nurses and more support workers. This trend offers great potential and attractions for nurses who are flexible and proactive. It implies the need for generic preparation leading to diplomas and degrees. People who cannot cope with, or do not want, a diploma or degree-level education can enter through the vocational qualifications route.

Variations on the main models

We developed two variants of the two main models.

The pragmatic model

As with the specialists, the pragmatists mourn the passing of specialist pre-registration courses leading to the Registered Mental Nurse (RMN) qualification but agree with the genericists that the trend is towards the generic nurse. In this situation DipHE courses represent the best chance that mental health nurses have of retaining their unique identity and specialist skills. What is important is to rein in the dominant influence of general nursing in the curricula of diploma courses so that the mental health branch can flourish. Unless this occurs nurses who select the pre-registration mental health branch are not given sufficient opportunity to develop the specialist skills valued by service managers. This state of affairs is self-defeating because it plays into the hands of nurses – mainly general nurses – who doubt the existence of specialist skills in mental health nursing. These doubters see these skills as simple variants on those used by all nurses in their psychosocial care of patients (see 'The unity-of-nursing model').

Pragmatists put emphasis on shoring up the boundaries of mental health nursing within the curriculum. Attempts to define and redefine the role of mental health nurses to reflect the nature of changing services (for example, *Working in Partnership*, DoH 1994) are welcomed. For pragmatists the therapeutic relationship between nurse and user is important, but it is no longer an adequate specification of the role and skills of the mental health nurse under the new service arrangements. Thus, for example, both case/care management as a form of service delivery and the orientation of services towards long-term mentally ill people, people with dual diagnoses and those with multiple disabilities have major implications for mental health nursing skills; and educational courses must adapt to meet them.

The structure and content of existing DipHE courses are crucial matters for pragmatists. They pay attention to the minutiae of curriculum planning, for example to the number of hours devoted to mental health nursing in the CFP, to the specialist nursing qualifications and experience of mental health nursing lecturers, and to the appointment of senior staff in colleges of nursing in higher education who have a background in and sympathy for the speciality.

The unity-of-nursing model

In common with the pragmatists, the unity-of-nursing model supports the current DipHE programmes but for rather different reasons. The unity-of-nursing model draws from the generic model the belief that there is nothing distinctive about the skills of mental health nurses compared with general nursing, which also addresses the psychosocial needs of patients. Shared learning is proposed across pre-registration branch programmes particularly for 'interpersonal skills', which emphasise therapeutic communication and humanistic counselling. Lecturers of these subjects are drawn from any nursing speciality, as long as they have an interest in psychosocial care and are skilled communicators. The specialist branch programme gives students the opportunity to practise these interpersonal and relationship skills in their chosen field. A key informant referred to these ideas as being part of a 'creeping colonisation' of mental health nursing by general nursing. This colonisation has occurred, she said, over the last 20 years as general nursing has embraced psychosocial care, so broadening its biomedical origins.

Popular mainly with general nurses, particularly those with a keen interest in psychosocial care, the unity-of-nursing model is criticised by specialists and pragmatists for simplifying the concept of nurse–patient (user) interpersonal communication. These critics argue that, for example, relating to a hallucinating and deluded person with a history of aggression requires a very different repertoire of interpersonal skills to those required to reassure an anxious person waiting for an operation. Proponents of the unity-of-nursing model are also criticised for holding to the concept of mental health nursing as centred on humanistic psychology, and for failing to take account of the influence of changing systems of service delivery on the role of the speciality.

Relevance of the models five years on

The study reported in this chapter was completed in the mid-1990s. What is the currency of the models of nurse education discussed here in the present context of mental health nursing in the UK? Clinical experience suggests that the genericist–specialist debate continues but that it has changed its character during this period. The study was concerned with the relationship between nursing specialities, in particular that between general (so-called Adult) nursing and the minority specialisms of mental health and learning disability nursing, within pre-registration DipHE programmes initiated by the Project 2000 reforms. This relationship was of great concern to mental health nurses in the early 1990s, but is, I think, of less concern to them today. There are, I suggest, two main reasons for this, both of which have increased once again the distance between mental health and general nursing, so reducing the likelihood of a generically prepared nurse. The first of these concerns UK pre-registration nursing reforms subsequent to the UKCC's Education Commission's report *Fitness for Practice* (UKCC 1999); the second concerns an increased emphasis on common training between health care professionals, particularly those working with specific patient groups. I comment on these issues below.

Repackaging UK pre-registration nursing programmes

In 2000 the UKCC revised the structure and organisation of the DipHE. This followed growing concern about the ability of these programmes to attract recruits to nursing in sufficient numbers and to produce nurses fit for practice (i.e. safe and competent practitioners) and for purpose (i.e. able to perform at the desired level – as required by managers and employers) at registration.

An assumption of the architects of Project 2000 and politicians of the day was that the initiative would improve recruitment to nursing and its professional status by locating nurse education in higher education. These expectations have not been fully realised, although without Project 2000 current recruitment might now be considerably worse. At the end of the 1990s the UK NHS was reported to be facing its worst shortage of qualified nurses in 25 years, and 80% of Trusts were experiencing 'medium to high problems in recruiting professional staff' (UKCC 1999). NHS staffing is still at the top of the political agenda. Two major government-led recruitment campaigns launched in early 1999 and in 2000 attracted considerable interest from those considering entering or returning to nursing. However, workforce analyses have shown that continuing demographic changes will mean that there will be fewer young people joining the workforce and more elderly people requiring longer-term care (Buchan & O'May 1998). The imperative therefore was to consider how pre-registration programmes could be repackaged to encourage more people to apply, and to accommodate recruits with different types of prior experience and knowledge.

The need for reform of pre-registration nurse education was also indicated by findings from several research studies that the DipHE was not preparing all students to meet the demands of practice at point of registration and beyond. There was concern, too, that the CFP was too long (18 months) and that it emphasised Adult Branch nursing and hospital-based care at the expense of the other branch programmes and community-based care (Jowett *et al.* 1994; While *et al.* 1995; Luker *et al.* 1996). What emerged from these research studies was a view that the attempt to eradicate the practice of student nurses being used as 'pairs of hands' in practice settings may have resulted in the pendulum swinging too far away from meeting service needs. They emphasised the importance of teachers and commissioners of pre-registration programmes working in a more collaborative way to ensure that future pre-registration nursing programmes would provide students with the ability to develop skills that would allow them to function effectively and with confidence in the workplace as registered practitioners.

These debates were taken forward in the UK government's white paper on nursing, *Making a Difference* (DoH 1999) and in the UKCC's Education Commission's report *Fitness for Practice* (UKCC 1999), which proposed a new model for pre-registration nurse education. The UKCC report reiterated the importance of striking a balance between theory and practice within the curriculum to ensure that students were fit for practice and for purpose on registration. DipHE programmes were perceived to have delayed students' direct experience with patients and as being over-theoretical. There were perceived problems too with the organisation and supervision of practice placements, which were compounded by pressure of work and the pace of activity in health care settings – factors that hinder, rather than facilitate, the development of practice skills. As a consequence, the sequencing and balance between college-based and practice-based study were recommended as a key area for review to ensure better integration of theory and practice (UKCC 1999). At the same time the UKCC report was clear in its recommendation that the number of graduate nurses must be increased to strengthen nursing leadership.

In September 1999 the UKCC accepted the recommendations of *Fitness for Practice* (UKCC 1999), with the result that new-styled pre-registration nursing programmes were introduced across the UK, with an initial tranche that started in England in September 2000. One of the most important changes was the introduction of a one-year (rather than 18-month) CFP which is taught in the context of all four branches, enables integration with the branch programmes and ensures that practice skills and placements are introduced at an early stage in the programme (UKCC 1999). These recommendations should reduce generic teaching within pre-registration nurse education and strengthen the identity of mental health nursing and other minority branch programmes.

Common core education across health care occupations

There will be new joint training across the professions in communication skills and in NHS principles and organisation. They will form part of a new core curriculum for all education programmes for NHS staff . . . A new common foundation programme will be put in place to enable students and staff to switch careers and training paths more easily. (DoH 2000a)

We believe it is important that the NHS . . . should work with higher education providers and accreditation bodies . . . to develop education and training arrangements which are genuinely multi-professional and which will enable students to transfer readily between courses without having to start their training afresh. (DoH 2000b)

These statements, taken from two major documents on the future of the UK NHS, demonstrate the central role now being accorded to multiprofessional and inter-professional education in the development of the 'new' NHS. Education for inter-professional working, as expressed here, implies at least four educational outcomes for students (Finch 2000). They need to:

(1) *know about* the roles of other professionals
(2) *be able to work with* other professionals in teams where each member has a clearly defined role
(3) *be able to substitute for* the roles of other professionals when circumstances suggest that this would be more effective
(4) *be able to move across* professional boundaries, so increasing career flexibility.

The capacity of higher education to meet *all* these objectives is uncertain, and how it might be accomplished is as yet unclear. It seems likely though that patient group or clinical speciality will be an increasingly important organising concept. For example, the Department of Health's review of the NHS workforce (DoH 2000b) proposed setting up Care Group Workforce Development Boards responsible for identifying changes and developments required in education and training to deliver a workforce with the skills required to support service changes in their specialist area, for example people suffering from mental illness.

One effect of these developments will be to broaden the generic–specialist debate within mental health nursing. This will involve consideration of the balance between core and discipline-specific education and training not simply with other nursing specialities, but also between the mental health nurses and other mental health care disciplines, including non-professionally trained workers. In the ascendant would seem to be what Rawson (1994) refers to as the 'melting-pot' model of inter-professional working in which professional groups have permeable boundaries offering potential for mutual transfer of elements. Rawson contrasts this with the 'mutual-respect' model in which professional boundaries are impermeable and inter-professional work remains subservient to the original occupational role of each professional group.

How mental health nurses will respond to these policy developments that support a common core training for health professionals is uncertain. However, as with the models of nurse education set out in this chapter, their response will be influenced greatly by their perception of mental health nursing as a practice discipline. Relevant here is the debate outlined by Repper (2000), between those mental health nurses who regard nursing as an 'art' and those who regard it as a 'science'. The former are primarily concerned with understanding mental health nursing as a discrete activity based on the relationship between the nurse and the individual *person* in *distress*, while the latter are primarily concerned with interventions or treatments (administered by nurses or others) for *patients* with a diagnosed mental *illness*. 'Specialists', the counterparts to 'artists' in the research outlined in this chapter, are likely to favour Rawson's (1994) mutual respect model of inter-professional working. They are also likely to favour a shift in balance in pre-registration curricula towards specialist preparation, designed to protect what they perceive to be the unique contribution of nursing to mental health care. Scientists, counterpart to our genericists, on the other hand, are more likely to favour the melting-pot model of inter-professional working, preparation for which would involve substantial core education across health care occupations.

Conclusion

The chapter has presented a picture of 'the field' from the perspective provided by ENB-funded research. It articulates interests including those of users and service consumers. The researchers at King's College aimed to identify the changing educational needs of mental health and learning disability nurses in the light of community care reforms, and found that perception of needs depends on how psychiatric nursing is seen, i.e. what model one has.

In conclusion, the models of nursing education espoused by respondents in the study reported here, and those that are likely to be endorsed in the future, are diverse. To some of the respondents in our study, the strong allegiance of some mental health nurses to one or other model, or to the artistic or scientific tradition, creates a disunited front which prevents the occupation from fashioning a coherent educational structure, particularly at pre-registration level. However, the debate between artists and scientists is not unique to mental health nursing. It is present in all practice disciplines and reflects differing research traditions (phenomenological vs. scientific) and differing views about what passes as knowledge. Such debates indicate a vibrant occupational group rather than one that is narrow and constrained in its thinking.

Whichever model or combination of models of nurse education is preferred, education providers face a complex challenge. The challenge is to produce mental health nurses able, on the one hand, to meet the needs of service users and the demands of service providers and, on the other hand, to maintain the standards of scholarship that higher education demands. The balance is not easy to achieve.

References

Altschul, A. (1964) Group dynamics and nursing care. *International Journal of Nursing Studies*, 1 (2): 151–8.

Buchan, J. & O'May, F. (1998) Nursing supply and demand: reviewing the evidence. *Nursing Times*, 94 (26): 60–63.

Department of Health (1994) *Working in Partnership: A Collaborative Approach to Care. Report of the Mental Health Nursing Review Team*. London: HMSO.

Department of Health (1999) *Making a Difference: Strengthening the Nursing, Midwifery and Health Visiting Contribution to Care*. London: DoH.

Department of Health (2000a) *The NHS Plan: A Plan for Investment, a Plan for Reform*. London: DoH.

Department of Health (2000b) *A Health Service of all the Talents: Developing the NHS Workforce*. London: DoH.

English National Board for Nursing, Midwifery and Health Visiting (1982) *Syllabus of Training: Professional Register – Part 3, Registered Mental Nurse*. London: ENB.

Finch, J. (2000) Inter-professional education and teamworking: a view from the education providers. *British Medical Journal*, 321: 1138–40.

Harries, C. (1978) Psychiatric nursing – therapists and beyond. In: *Contemporary Themes in Psychiatric Nursing* (ed. H. Leopoldt). Twickenham, Middlesex: Squibb & Sons.

Jones, J. & Jones, D. (1992) Education for the future: meeting challenging needs. In: *Project 2000: The Teachers Speak* (eds O. Slevin & M. Buckingham). London: Campion Press.

Jowett, S., Walton, I. & Payne, S. (1994) *Challenges and Change in Nurse Education – A Study of the Implementation of Project 2000*. Slough: National Foundation for Education Research.

Luker, K., Carlisle, C., Davis, C., Riley, E., Stilwell, J. & Watson, R. (1996) *Project 2000. Fitness for Practice*. Liverpool: Joint Report of the Universities of Liverpool and Warwick to the DoH.

Mangan, P. (1992) Pruning back. *Nursing Times*, 88 (50): 18–19.

Ministry of Health (1968) *Psychiatric Nursing Today and Tomorrow*. London: HMSO.

Nolan, P. & Hopper, B. (2000) Revisiting mental health nursing in the 1960s. *Journal of Mental Health*, 9 (6): 563–73.

Norman, I.J. (1998a) The changing emphasis of mental health and learning disability nurse education in the UK and ideal models of its future development. *Journal of Psychiatric and Mental Health Nursing*, 5: 41–51.

Norman, I.J. (1998b) Priorities for mental health and learning disability nurse education in the UK: a case study. *Journal of Clinical Nursing*, 7: 433–41.

Norman, I.J. & Redfern, S.J. with Bodley, D., Holroyd, S., Smith, C. & White, E. (1996) *The changing educational needs of mental health and learning disability nurses*. Project report to the English National Board for Nursing, Midwifery and Health Visiting. London: ENB.

Peplau, H. (1952) *Interpersonal Relations in Nursing*. New York: G.P. Putman.

Rawson, D. (1994) Models of interprofessional work: likely theories and possibilities. In: *Going Inter-professional: Working Together for Health and Welfare* (ed. A. Leathard). London: Routledge.

Repper, J. (2000) Adjusting the focus of mental health nursing: incorporating service users' experiences of recovery. *Journal of Mental Health*, 9 (6): 575–87.

Royal College of Nursing (1985) *The Education of Nurses: A New Dispensation*. Judge Report. London: RCN.

Royal College of Nursing (1993) *Evidence to the National Review of Mental Health Nursing*. London: RCN.

Samson, C. (1995) The fracturing of medical dominance in British psychiatry? *Sociology of Health and Illness*, 17 (2): 245–68.

Thomas, B. (1992) Education. In: *A Textbook of Psychiatric and Mental Health Nursing* (eds J. Brooking, S. Ritter & B. Thomas). Edinburgh: Churchill Livingstone.

Thomas, B. (1993) A dilution of skills. *Nursing Times*, 89 (29): 30–31.

United Kingdom Central Council for Nursing, Midwifery and Health Visiting (1986) *Project 2000: A New Preparation for Practice*. London: UKCC.

United Kingdom Central Council for Nursing, Midwifery and Health Visiting (1999) *Fitness for Practice: Report of the UKCC Commission for Education* (Chair: Sir Len Peach). London: UKCC.

Weller, M (1989) Mental illness – who cares? *Nature*, 339: 249–52.

While, A.E., Roberts, J. & Fitzpatrick, J. (1995) *A Comparative Study of Outcomes of Pre-registration Nurse Education Programmes*. London: Department of Nursing Studies, King's College London.

White, E., Riley, E., Davies, S. & Twinn, S. (1993) *A detailed study of the relationships between teaching, support, supervision and role modelling in clinical areas, within the context of Project 2000 courses*. Report to the ENB, King's College London and University of Manchester.

Yin, R.K. (1989) *Case Study Research: Design and Methods*. Newbury Park: Sage.

Section 3

Analytic and Critical Commentaries and Conclusion

Chapter 9

Reflective Commentaries by the Contributors to Section 2: Each Sees the Field from Within the Field

Commentary 9.1
Much in Common: Relationships and Knowledge in the Developing Field

Kevin Gournay

Since writing my contribution for Section 2 there have been major developments in mental health policy in England and it is likely that similar developments will follow in other parts of the UK. These changes have, in a sense, overshadowed my reading of the contributions from colleagues. Recently the most important event has been the setting up of the National Institute for Mental Health for England (NIMHE), which the government sees as a way of ensuring that, first of all, mental health services are developed strategically and with equity across England, and, second, resources are used most effectively to develop education, training and research. England now has regional centres for NIMHE which will focus on service development and education and training. The second major initiative is the setting up of a research network, using a hub and spoke model. The hub of the NIMHE research network is formed by the Health Services Research Department (with other colleagues) at the Institute of Psychiatry and the Department of Psychiatry in the University of Manchester. The key members of the hub include psychiatrists, psychologists, nurses, social workers and service user researchers, with considerable support from various other colleagues. Eventually, the spokes will reach out to the key research centres across the country and it is envisaged that research studies will, in future, become multi-centred and representative in terms of their samples. There are a number of other important initiatives related to NIMHE, including the building of an infrastructure to support education and training and policy development, as well as new initiatives to assist with improving the capacity of research oriented departments by increasing skills at various levels across all of the relevant disciplines. Although devolution has of course brought a great diversity across the four countries of the UK, there is no doubt that Scotland, Wales and Northern Ireland will employ similar initiatives to ensure comprehensive, strategic and cost-effective approaches to service development, education and training, and research.

The other major change in policy, which has more direct implications for nursing, is the dissolution of the United Kingdom Central Council for Nursing, Midwifery and Health Visiting, and the setting up of the Nursing and Midwifery Council (NMC). This new body has an entirely different way of including lay members and, with major changes such as the emphasis on the concept of fitness for practice, may well lead to substantial changes in nursing practice. However, while the setting up of the NMC is important, it is, perhaps, not so relevant to this chapter and I will not provide further discussion here. Suffice it to say that this and other changes in policy continue apace and, as a consequence, changes in health care will be substantial.

Finally, although it is only a few months since I finished my first contribution to this book, I have to note the gathering pace of the implementation of an evidence-based approach to health care, particularly in the field of mental health. It has now become clear that many of the therapies and approaches that lacked an evidence base and which are nevertheless widespread across the country are now in steep decline. The National Service Framework and the principles under-pinning NIMHE emphasise the requirement to deliver services that are based wherever possible on the rigorous evidence that comes from randomised control-led trials. As a corollary of this, the National Institute for Clinical Excellence (NICE) is now in the midst of producing evidence-based guidance for a number of conditions and approaches, including recently schizophrenia.

How, then, do all these changes make me see the contributions of my col-leagues? I suppose my first thought is that, with regard to the above areas, much of what was written by my colleagues seems to have been done without any consideration of more general major policy developments that have occurred in each and every part of the UK since 1997. However, that said, there is a clear acknowledgement by my colleagues that the nature of mental health nursing is undergoing tremendous change. If I were to identify the most important area raised in the various contributions by my colleagues, I would cite that of user and carer involvement, described by Forrest and Masters. Although they have only identified issues relating to mental health nursing education, rather than mental health care generally, they have quite rightly pointed to the difficulties involved in ensuring that users and carers are involved in every stage of the process from beginning of curriculum design, through to actual delivery. The relevance to 'the field of knowledge' is absolutely clear. Through their chapter, Forrest and Masters have demonstrated that, when we look at what mental health nursing is, and how it develops, we have to see a collaborative approach between nurses and users and carers as paramount. Arguably, the spirit of collaboration is demonstrated in modern mental health nursing in the practice of cognitive beha-viour therapy, helping patients deal with the difficulties of taking medications – which on the one hand may alleviate some of their distress and suffering, but on the other hand can produce major problems – through motivational inter-viewing approaches, and more generally in the way that skilled mental health nurses now develop care plans with rather than for the patient.

Norman's chapter provides a great deal of food for thought about the different approaches to nursing education. However, in citing his very carefully executed research, funded by the English National Board, he describes an initiative of yesteryear. English National Board-commissioned research is now replaced by the research programmes of NIHME, the Medical Research Council and other funding bodies, which, of course, all function in the new era of research govern-ance, with all its attendant processes of transparency, equity and improved ethical underpinning. Also, it is clear that the idea of funding pure 'mental health nursing research' is now a thing of the past. The departments of health in the four countries of the UK are now focusing on topics of importance that form a common agenda for all professions and users and carers. These include areas where nursing is central, such as inpatient care, but the research process and, in turn, the contribution to 'the field of knowledge' should now be seen much more generically. Similarly, research training for nurses is now clearly part of the multidisciplinary endeavour to improve capacity, rather than an isolated approach. Norman highlights the differences in approach to mental health nursing education which are demonstrated in the chapters of this book.

In conclusion, I feel that my fellow contributors and I have much in common. All of my colleagues have emphasised that, whatever the arguments regarding our view of 'the field of knowledge', it is the relationship between the nurse and the patient that is of central importance. From my reading of the contributions by my colleagues, our field of knowledge seems at the moment to comprise scientific and non-scientific approaches and I am left with the view that mental health nursing would be much poorer if one or the other influence was missing.

Commentary 9.2
On Readings on the Field

Stephen Tilley

I will interpret the field of knowledge, based on reading my co-contributors' chapters, as a site for display of 'goods internal to' the fragile tradition's scholarly practice:

(1) challenging psychiatric and mental health nurses (PMHNs) to account for (and argue about) nursing practice in professional, policy and institutional contexts
(2) challenging them to change their practices in light of (1)
(3) challenging the basis of relationships in practice.

The chapters fall into two clusters. Chapters 2, 4 and 8 I read as challenging PMHNs to *account for* practice on the basis of (more or less) institutionally secure field-constructing knowledge. By contrast, Chapters 5, 6 and 7 challenge PMHNs to *argue about* practice on the basis of (more or less) institutionally insecure knowledge which challenges dominant knowledge. Those in the two clusters do not argue directly *with each other*: I have to *imagine* the argument that might take place between them, to sustain *my sense* of the field as tradition-informed (and the tradition of field-shaping). I will differentiate the two clusters, then consider the conditions for *realisation* of that field.

Challenging PMHNs to account (and argue) in professional, policy and institutional contexts

The accounts of institutionalised knowledge differ in how they challenge PMHNs to account in professional, policy and institutional contexts. Gournay, Griffiths and Franks, and Norman challenge PMHNs by representing their own institutions' forms of knowledge as *constructing* the field; Carson, Forrest and Masters, and Chambers *et al.* challenge PMHNs by representing theirs as *challenging dominant constructions* of the field.

In Chapter 2, Gournay presents the Institute's knowledge as multiprofessional, evidence-based and service-delivery focused, and highly integrated. These are also presented as the characteristics of the field structured by policy and by professional and institutional power. PMHNs are challenged to take a 'truly multidisciplinary approach to the problems of modern mental health care' and develop knowledge pertaining to the nursing *function* within mental health services. In Chapter 4, Griffiths and Franks present an account of a 'new discipline' and 'meta-paradigm' for PMHNing stemming from the 'culture of inquiry' at the Cassel Hospital and shaped by application of the 'Tavistock discourse' to nursing. Through struggles to institutionalise this 'new discipline' they are able to 'position this field of knowledge and practice within the wider field of mental health nursing, nursing and developments more generally within the health care system'. In Chapter 8, Norman summarises research that formulated models of the PMHN as 'specialists' or 'generalists' (or variants). He further interprets these models in the context of developments in multi-professional, patient-group focused education in the ' "new" NHS', and in terms of Rawson's more general account of inter-professional working.

By contrast to these field-constructing accounts, Carson presents himself (Chapter 5) as working in a *'corner* of the field' (italics added), where he subjects to self-reflective analysis a curriculum promoting practice as application of context-free and abstract knowledge. Thereby he challenges PMHNs to practise instead under the auspices of the principle of respecting people's wholeness 'that should always be part of practice in the field that is mental health nursing'. For Carson, even when the field is regulated by policy or professional authority, principled practice is necessarily always local and contextualised, based on relationship with whole persons. In Chapter 6, Forrest and Masters recount their response to policy promoting user involvement: involving users to develop a curriculum for mental health nurses. This took them 'toward a version of mental health nursing' that values human qualities more highly than professional qualities. This in turn challenged their sense of professional personal identity and their relationships with academic colleagues. In Chapter 7, Chambers *et al.* challenged each other to 'write across differences'; differences of personal and impersonal knowledge and differences in their positions inside/outside institutions. Their knowledge challenges other knowledges that separate reason and unreason.

In all the latter three chapters, the authors construct their knowledges for practice *in* the field as won through challenge of what they portray as a dominant construction *of* the field. Carson discerns care as essential to PMHN practice, 'therapeutic involvement' as subject to discretion; Forrest and Masters endorse human qualities as primary in PMHNing, balanced with professional qualities; Chambers *et al.* assert the priority of individualisation over institutionalisation. Thus, the less institutionally secure knowledges (in Chapters 5, 6 and 7) provide accounts of 'other' practice-guiding knowledge claims and, through their own knowledge-work resist them: recovering the good through self-reflection (Carson), refusing to rule out or keep out the other's knowledge (Forrest and Masters); challenging discrimination (Chambers *et al.*).

This contrasts with the way the 'other' knowledge is addressed in accounts of the more institutionally secure knowledges (Chapters 2, 4 and 8). For example, Gournay addresses mental health nurses who would participate in this framework:

We obviously need to continue with our attempts to develop a theoretical understanding of what components of mental health nursing are effective. Simply put, it is our view that we should start almost with a tabula rasa and cast aside various archaic theories which continue to preoccupy many nursing academics and which are merely a source of frustration. (p. 28)

Such erasure or casting aside of knowledge that frustrates one's knowledge-constructing project is the epistemological inverse of Carson's method of self-reflection as the basis of principled practice (which requires close attention to the implications of an 'other's' claims). Again, Norman's construction of mental health nursing in terms of inter*professional* relationships does not provide a basis for recognising the epistemological challenge posed by Chambers *et al.*'s claims for the authority of experiential knowledge. Furthermore, in Griffiths and Franks' paradigm, users' knowledge will always appear as interpreted through the lens of systemic and psychodynamic understandings.

The field and the tradition

What, according to this reading, is needed if the field in which we *all* regard each other – which *none* can see from outside the field – is to be a site for scholarly practice in the fragile tradition? The goods of the fragile tradition would best be realised in *this* field if all accepted and fulfilled the obligation of *collective* accountability for challenging and being open to challenge from each other. For those more institutionally secure this entails a correlative challenge of responsibility – proportionate to their power – to test the authority of their knowledges in direct argument with 'others'.

Commentary 9.3
Are All as One Among Many and of Equal Value?

Peter Griffiths and Vicky Franks

A more important consideration, in our opinion, is the value that each field brings to mental health nursing and the capacity of each to strengthen the practice of mental health nurse education. Ian Norman's study of models of mental health nursing (Chapter 8) is particularly relevant now because of concerns about the future place of mental health nursing and the rise of the non-professionally aligned mental health worker. We were left with the question: What does mental health nursing practice have to offer which is unique? We believe the answer lies in the collaborative relationships that mental health nurses develop with colleagues, patients and carers. This has to be based on a sound understanding of biomedical and psychosocial knowledge. Our field occupies the psychosocial domain. We describe below our perception of this domain and how it fits with the larger field of mental health nursing, and conclude with some thoughts about the relative balance with other domains in the field.

Therapeutic involvement

Ian Norman says that supporters of the specialist model believe that 'the exercise of the nurse's therapeutic relationship is most vividly expressed in his or her capacity to stick with and maintain relationships with long-term seriously ill people'. We would describe this as our position and so it seems would many of the other contributors. Alexander McMurdo Carson (Chapter 5) makes a sound argument for an ethical framework based on the holistic nature of people and, in accord with psychoanalytic thinking, does not separate the psyche from the soma. He believes there is a close relationship between therapeutic involvement and clinical competence. This is reminiscent of Steve Tilley's account of his students and the tradition in which he works. A large part of Alexander's chapter focuses on therapeutic involvement; he calls this the language game distinctive to mental health nursing.

What is therapeutic involvement?

The assumption we make when teaching within our paradigm is that, as Susanne Forrest and Hugh Masters say in Chapter 6, patients require practitioners to be 'in touch with their own mental distress and vulnerability'. Thus the nurse needs to be emotionally affected by the patient if he or she is going to be therapeutic. To return to Alexander's chapter, we diverge from his position in two ways. First, we do not believe that 'therapy is a defence against getting too close and being overwhelmed by feeling'. Indeed, the use of a therapeutic framework like psychoanalytic theory enables nurses to acknowledge and examine the emotions evoked by the patient and to think about them without being overwhelmed and acting on them prematurely. Second, what Alexander describes as therapy we would be more likely to describe as therapeutic involvement. In our framework this means that the practical problems, which he separates from therapy, as he calls it, would and could be two faces of therapeutic work. This last point underlies the Cassel model of psychosocial nursing, which emphasises the therapeutic potential of everyday activities within a therapeutically-informed environment.

The hazards of therapeutic involvement

Susanne and Hugh describe and defend a user-led curriculum. Work in our paradigm has traditionally not involved users to the extent that it might. It is probably because our thinking examines the patient's unconscious impulse to sabotage help, and the particularly destructive nature of some patients who, because of specific personality characteristics, are prone to reject and subvert all relationships. The field in which we work emphasises the nature of the transference/countertransference and the extent to which patients behave towards the professional as if the latter were another person in the patient's life. Thus we acknowledge the difficulty in being rational with patients who feel, think and behave in irrational ways. Patients can affect staff through objective countertransference as well as through subjective countertransference responses stimulated in staff due to their own pasts. However, we do think we could involve patients and their carers more, in order to work with and engender positive connection, 'to care with' rather than 'to care for' patients, as Susanne and Hugh say. At the Cassel this is called 'working alongside'. We sound a note of caution with regard to the excellent work described by Susanne and Hugh, however, in relation to the effect of breaking down the professional/user/patient boundary. They indicate the powerful effect of this on users; in our parlance, we would say that the users feel less split off and constructed as different and aberrant. However, sometimes splits can be protective. If the institution is not structured around this way of working, then the students and the few committed lecturers may be left feeling very exposed.

In defence of therapeutic involvement

Most of the chapters acknowledged the large part emotional involvement plays in mental health nursing, and the use of something variously described as common sense, tacit knowledge or unconscious communication. The relative value placed on this knowledge and the evidence of the emotions is contested in Kevin Gournay's chapter (Chapter 2). He makes a strong case for randomised controlled trials (RCTs) and believes that arguments against them are largely vacuous. We believe that it is not possible to research all aspects of the work of mental health professionals by that means. Indeed, the findings from RCTs are based on samples of populations (to allow generalisation) and we believe that for mental health nurses this does not capture the unique nature of the nurse/patient relationship. To grasp at certainties in the form of RCTs is to deny the problem of fallibility. A psychoanalytic writer, Edna O'Shaugnessy, makes a very simple but pertinent point in these days of risk management, namely that all human knowledge is known through the distorting frame of the human mind (O'Shaugnessy 1994). The human mind is not wholly rational and we are more likely to make mistakes if we are fearful of feelings like doubt and uncertainty. The professional's tacit (unconscious) knowledge can be researched, though not by using RCTs.

The balance between scientific rationality and therapeutic intuition

Kevin's chapter is impressive and broad, covering vast areas of importance, but there is a sense of the field being more important than the modest aims of relationship building in nursing. The biomedical model dominates mental health nursing. There needs to be a balance between sound evidence-based, biologically and pharmaceutically informed practice and emotionally engaged practice. We (in the psychosocial domain) need Kevin's field as much as he needs ours, but we need to get our house in order. We believe that the field of therapeutically informed mental health nursing as it is represented here can be confusing and too theoretical. We know that we psychoanalytically informed teachers are sometimes guilty of too much theorising and of using esoteric language. We were struck as we read some chapters by our struggle to engage with the ideas because they were steeped in such dense and specialist language. Is it any wonder then that our students grasp at the more concrete facts of biomedicine? Alexander expects his diploma-level students to be critical and analytical thinkers. This is difficult enough for Steve Tilley's BSc and postgraduate students. We are not sure where this leaves our field except that we need to make our paradigm more accessible. In keeping with our tradition we need to examine our own sense of omnipotence and learn to explain our ideas without recourse to impressive jargon.

Reference

O'Shaugnessy, E. (1994) What is a clinical test? *International Journal of Psychoanalysis*, 75: 939–47.

Commentary 9.4
Re-searching Practice: A Critical Conversation

Alexander McMurdo Carson

The conversation that was constructed in these first chapters displays a number of understandings about what mental health nursing really is. However, these understandings are articulated in exclusive ways. To some extent these chapters seem like monologues rather than parts in a real conversation. Real conversation makes room for the other, while some of these papers explicitly or implicitly resist any view but their own. Gournay, for example, wants to resist any conversation with other practitioners who hold different views on the value of other research methodologies. Other papers offer resistance to a medical view of mental illness and privilege direct experience. Each monologue understands itself as an authentic and valuable version of mental health nursing. The value of these differences is assumed rather than articulated, and when we scratch below the surfaces these differences are more apparent than real. While these different views seem like real differences, these *different* views are not really so different. All privilege knowledge or know-how, whether it is techniques like randomised controlled trials or 'involvement'. However, the impression given in these chapters is that the field of knowledge has developed historically and randomly in a way that does seem to make the tradition look fragile and constantly in a state of flux. What this field as tradition and conversation is lacking is a method or way of developing an authentic conversation among knowledge claimants in the field, rather than a series of unconnected monologues. The practitioners and authors that constitute the field of knowledge are engaged in what Heidegger (1962) calls 'idle talk'; that is, conversation that has no foundations and simply drifts along. What the field of knowledge needs in order to develop this conversation is a more authentic 'other'; something other than knowledge. In this short section, I propose to review the first chapters as a conversation that could be developed. In developing this conversation I am guided by Arendt's warning:

> If it should turn out to be true that knowledge (in the modern sense of know-how) and thought have parted company for good, then we would indeed become the helpless slaves, not so much of our machines as of our know-how, thoughtless creatures at the mercy of every gadget which is technically possible. . . . (Arendt 1989: 3)

Arendt points to the need to develop a conversation between reflection and knowledge because the consequence of not doing so might be that knowledge alone comes to define the field. The result could be that the field continues to drift along without any clear identity. I will begin with a review of these chapters and what they say about mental health nursing and will conclude with a suggestion about a possible way forward.

Mental health nursing as know-how

These first chapters display a number of ways of seeing the field of knowledge. For Gournay, the position is clear. Gournay's chapter considers mental health nursing's field of knowledge to be too fragile to be sustained without help from partners such as psychiatry, although not general nursing, to build a 'mental health community'. His practice is the 'input–output' model where success can be measured objectively in the amount of grant capture and Research Assessment Exercise scores. Gournay considers any other model of practice to be dubious and sees any further conversation as 'vacuous'. He also wants to resist any further questioning or evaluation as he thinks that 'only time will tell' if he is right.

Forrest and Masters take the opposite point of view. They are less sure than Gournay concerning what mental health nursing is about, but they are certainly against the valuing of objective knowledge in the way that Gournay proposes. Rather than see mental health nursing as constituted by medical intervention, they want to resist this instrumental approach by proposing that personal involvement should be the practice of choice. In a similar way, Griffiths and Franks base their practice in the tradition that they inherited from the Tavistock Clinic. At the heart of this practice is the notion of practitioners as knowledge producers, which they believe can help clients to develop. They subscribe to the standard of sincerity in practice.

Both Chambers *et al.* and Tilley see mental health nursing as being constituted by strong individuals. Tilley shows the conversation among pioneers that has constituted the tradition of mental health nursing at his institution. He wants to suggest that mental health nursing can develop if teachers, researchers and practitioners become more conscious or thoughtful about their practice/accounts. Chambers *et al.* want to value the role that 'strong individuals' can play in the development of mental health nursing. They think that experiential knowledge can be a valuable resource that can transform learning about mental distress and lead to a 'just peace'. This too is a chapter that wants value to be given to the suffering and distress that users experience.

What is really missing from these accounts is any sense that the field can develop in better ways rather than just different ways. Part of the reason for this is that the potential conversation has no strong standard or developmental thread that can sustain or develop the conversation and thus the field. The authors who support a less objective, professional development of the field are not really engaging with authors such as Gournay; they are just proposing a more subjective, personal approach. What the field or conversation needs to develop is something more than monologues about know-how. To develop the field would require the laying of firmer foundations, and my chapter in these first chapters suggests that a more serious and respectful engagement between authors and practitioners could do this.

Reflection in the field of knowledge

I approached the construction of my narrative as an outsider who wanted to engage with the inside. I trained as a general nurse and, apart from an eight-week placement in a large psychiatric institution, have no experience of mental health nursing. I began my engagement by taking seriously the claims made about mental health nursing in a mental health curriculum. I made the assumption that the standard that mental health nursing is guided by would be there in the curriculum as practice. I showed that while the curriculum, as theory, proposed to respect people as whole persons, the curriculum, as practice, valued therapeutic knowledge more. I suggested that this version of mental health nursing practice was a mistake and I suggested that respect for clients as whole persons should determine, situation by situation, the appropriateness of applied knowledge. In the larger context provided by the chapters in the previous section, this seems all the more necessary.

On reading these chapters, I am left with the impression that this field of knowledge is constantly changing and taking on board whatever the latest technique or know-how is. What is missing from the field is any criterion for evaluating new knowledge. Of course we cannot develop criteria for judging the admissibility of new knowledge to the field, from within that knowledge itself. I am suggesting that mental health nursing should develop its field in a more thoughtful way by remembering what it is really all about; helping people who are suffering and need our help. This is not something that is new but something that was, in reality, always a part of the field but often remained unrecognized and undervalued.

Conclusion

The field of mental health nursing will develop when researchers, educators and practitioners recognize the value of different approaches to suffering and distress. While both subjective and objective forms of knowledge have constituted the field historically, this jostling has led to an unstable or fragile tradition. Rather than value new knowledge because of its difference, mental health nursing's field of knowledge needs to learn to evaluate this difference. To do this requires recognition of the ethical foundations in which it is located.

References

Arendt, H. (1989) *The Human Condition*. Chicago: University of Chicago Press.
Heidegger, M. (1962) *Being and Time*. Oxford: Blackwell.

Commentary 9.5
Field of Knowledge: A Critical Commentary

Hugh Masters and Susanne Forrest

Before considering the various contributors' accounts of the field of psychiatric and mental health nursing it is perhaps important to note that current discourses about mental health nursing (evident in policy documents, practice accounts and recent literature) suggest a profession with disparate accounts of what it is about and what its future direction should be. After reading the various chapters, it is apparent that there is some degree of consensus among contributors regarding the aspirations and future directions for the profession. These appear to centre on three intertwined areas: '(re)humanising' mental health nursing; service user involvement as a means to achieve this; and reinterpreting and challenging the current interpretations of evidence-based health care.

Perhaps it is also worth considering that this book is not '*the* field of knowledge' but represents areas of the field and a collection of views of certain individuals in certain institutions. How widespread these views are is open to question. Importantly the extent to which these opinions actually influence or seem relevant to practitioners, or impact on mental health nursing practice, also needs to be honestly considered. The accounts show that the foundations and traditions that have shaped the individual institutions' approaches to mental health nursing education and research are diverse. Griffiths and Franks, Tilley, and Gournay are able to demonstrate, and draw on, particular traditions in their respective institutions. It is apparent, however, that in the other accounts there is much less of a sense of a tradition. Rather, contributors describe a history of adapting and 'borrowing' from the traditions of other academic disciplines, usually without satisfaction and resolution, in their attempts to define and make sense of the role of the mental health nurse. They are now perhaps borrowing from, or at least aligning themselves with, the traditions and values of the service user/survivor movements. This highlights the disparate and (as Tilley notes) often-fragile traditions in which mental health nursing is rooted. It would be interesting to revisit these accounts in 10 years time to see if user involvement has proved to be a more durable, defining force than, for example, the predecessors such as psychoanalysis, humanism, sociology, psychology and psychiatry.

When readers view the accounts as a whole, there will be a sense of disbelief at how many words and arguments are presented to state, and restate, the well-rehearsed argument that the person and not the disease should be central to mental health nursing. It may also seem extraordinary that the centrality of listening to people's stories and accounts in a human, warm, personal and empathic way needs to be argued (or indeed is open to argument). So why have so many of the authors felt the need to state these arguments? In almost all the accounts there is obvious widespread discontent with the standard of current mental health services, the dominance of psychiatry and the emphasis on disease. It is argued within the chapters that psychiatry still devalues people's experiences and narratives, and converts them into signs and symptoms which fit into predefined diagnostic criteria. Psychiatry is vilified as the force that militates against seeing people as valued individuals who have expertise about their own mental health. In relation to this it is apparent that the language in the 'field' is still difficult, confused and culturally loaded. Keen (2003), in an eloquent discussion of the relationship between psychiatry and nursing, sees two questions as central: will nursing continue to align itself with psychiatry; and will we be seen as 'psychiatric nurses' (or instead as more autonomous and psychosocially orientated 'mental health nurses'). Whilst the accounts generally accord with the notion of 'mental health nurses', Gournay shows a tradition, and a future, aligned to psychiatry and its values and knowledge. Interestingly none of the authors questions in any depth whether mental health nursing as a profession actually has a future or whether a generic Mental Health Worker may supersede all the arguments and viewpoints proposed.

The current and prominent policy of evidence-based health care and the difficulties of this policy in terms of the push and pull it exerts on gathering and using 'evidence' within mental health nursing education is at the forefront of many of the accounts. There is broad agreement about the need to find a way to value people's accounts about their experiences of mental health, distress, illness and services within the framework of evidence. However, the difficulties of writing about experience, as described by Forrest and Masters and Chambers *et al.*, may give a clue to the difficulties of discussing this 'evidence' objectively. The similarities in the paths taken in these two chapters are notable. Similar processes of attempting to write personal accounts of involvement and experience of mental distress led to considerable stalling, followed by a period of trying to reconcile what these accounts meant in terms of knowledge and evidence. The ultimate realisation was that it was the reflexive process that was crucial, rather than the actual experiences and outcomes. Chambers *et al.* note that 'integrating knowledge about the human experience of crisis, loss, mental distress, mental illness (however we wish to describe it) into the curriculum of health and social care professionals will necessarily be fraught with difficulty'. That said, arguably the most enlightening and powerful accounts about academics' viewpoints, and what has shaped them, are to be found in the personal accounts contained within the chapter by Chambers *et al.* Perhaps the one chapter that does not share this view (or does not do so overtly) is that by Gournay. Here the emphasis is very much on psychiatric nursing rather than mental health nursing. Gournay argues that research should only gather and value users' views and experiences if these can be used directly in demonstrating measurable outcomes of care in 'high quality' research (essentially, research based on the randomised controlled trial). User views are relegated to the status of data-source rather than being seen as the foundation of care.

The call for the adoption of the policy of user involvement in education is powerful within the chapters overall. This approach is seen as a way to build relationships with individual users of services and user organisations, but, most importantly, as the way in which the agenda of humanising education and care is legitimised. Whilst the chapters clearly show that most contributors have embraced the ubiquitous policy of user involvement, questions about how it will be implemented remain. The move to custodial and social control in the draft English Mental Health Act (and perhaps to a lesser extent the emerging Scottish Act, passed in 2003) and the current vogue of 'competency'-based education may conflict with the philosophy of involvement and joint working. Additionally, will user involvement mirror the implementation of student involvement in higher education curricula, which as Chambers *et al.* note is very much a marginal activity, with at best tokenistic consultation and little or no student power? Or will it mirror service user involvement in practice and become more rhetoric than reality, or politically correct tokenism rather than actual involvement?

Reference

Keen, T. (2003) Post-psychiatry: paradigm shift or wishful thinking? A speculative review of future possibilities for psychiatry. *Journal of Psychiatric and Mental Health Nursing*, 10 (1): 29–37.

Commentary 9.6
Knowledge Camps and Difference: Critical Exploration in the Field

Mary Chambers and Tessa Parkes

Reading the seven chapters for this book was a stimulating task. In this commentary we will comment on two key themes that emerged from our reflection and discussion on the content of these varied contributions. The themes are *knowledge camps* and *making sense of difference*.

Knowledge camps

Each chapter seemed unique in terms of content, contribution to knowledge and writing style; yet a certain synergy existed across a number of them. Such individuality and diversity adds to the overall appeal and value of the book with respect to our understanding of the state-of-the-art of nursing knowledge. However, this also raised more questions than it provided answers, questions such as: What do we have in common? Are there any core values or core knowledges? Where does this leave users? How do we make sense of this as educators to new recruits in mental health nursing? How does this fit with practice 'on the ground'?

It was interesting for each of us to realise how emotional were our reactions to each of the pieces of writing. We found it easy to identify with some pieces and hard to value or appreciate others, largely because of our own positions within the field but also because of features of writing and language that made us unwilling to engage with the arguments. Reading the chapters provoked feelings of frustration, confusion, relief and comfort as we identified, or did not identify, with the content and style of each of the pieces.

Overall there was a sense that there were 'knowledge camps' in that some chapters seemed to fit together well, e.g. complementary with some shared core assumptions, whereas others seemed to speak from positions that appeared oppositional to other chapters because they seemed to lie in different camps. The chapters arguably represent a polarisation of fields and forms of knowledge, with some favouring a more positivist approach and others an experiential one; largely, with little in between.

The 'positivist' work represents the use of deduction as a means of knowledge generation and this is reflected in the methodology of randomised controlled trials with statistically determined outcomes. No explicit credence or value is given to the importance of personal experience and its associated knowledge; quite the opposite, in fact, where a narrow concern with professionally and politically identified notions of effectiveness and positive outcomes leads to a lack of critical reflection on alternative visions and voices. To our minds such methodologies are surely limited in a discipline such as nursing, which is concerned with the nature of mental distress as experienced by individuals, in that they do little to facilitate an understanding of individual responses to mental illness. However, in the current political climate this methodology is considered the 'gold standard' of research, despite many such studies being seriously flawed as a result of different types of bias.

We have an affinity with experiential and personal forms of knowledge, as we outline in our collective chapter. This makes us sympathetic to chapters that also value these sources and forms of knowledge and their associated methodologies. In our view the chapters utilising a more experiential approach give greater insight into the experience of mental illness/distress and its consequences for individuals, families and communities. Whilst understanding the importance of knowledge diversity, as mental health nurses, academics and teachers we hesitate to embrace forms of knowledge – such as the positivist approach advocated in the Institute of Psychiatry chapter (Chapter 2) – oppositional to further embracing and moving towards experiential knowledge forms.

Although there is an increasing acceptance of the value of experiential knowledge, it is clear from the chapters addressing nurse education that much has yet to be achieved before it can have its rightful place at the centre of the curriculum.

Nursing curricula can often adhere to formalised knowledge and teaching methods, reinforcing the medical model and perpetuating the divide between service users and professionals. In these cases we believe that nursing students continue to be exposed to nursing knowledge and skills in a mechanistic manner, which impacts on their socialisation and works against the development of an inquiring and critical approach. Experiential knowledge, as considered here and in our chapter, is about an individual's interpretation of the lived experience of mental illness/distress. It is impossible to transmit such knowledge in the traditional manner described above and it is our view that a greater appreciation of the challenges of how to address this within the curricula would have enhanced the overall contribution of this book to nursing knowledge.

Making sense of difference

So in the light of the above, how do we make sense of the different contributions to this timely book? Is it a problem that there are such polar views? Is it necessary to have a consensus on key values, knowledges and associated competencies in mental health nursing? Does it matter that such an array of versions of mental illness/distress exists in our practices, curricula, research and in our writing about these activities? We are not sure. It strikes us as a potentially bewildering situation both for users and carers and for nursing students, who need to navigate through this territory from relatively weak positions of power and authority. There are clearly strengths in the diversity of the knowledge bases from which we can draw, but perhaps we need to be working to find more commonalties than exist at present, rather than staying wedded to our own intellectual 'comfort zones'. Maybe others of us writing here have ideas about how we can make sense of all our differences or pull together some core threads that can be said to be representative of mental health nursing knowledge in the UK.

The diversity of approaches contained within this book could and should act as a springboard and catalyst for a more collective, critical exploration of the nature of knowledge and its transmission, pertinent to future generations of health care professionals. We would like to see more exploration with users and carers of the forms and fields of knowledge that seem most useful and valuable for them, with a view to making mental health nursing practice more sensitive to their needs and wants. Placing the experiential knowledge of individuals at the core of all our activities could be one way to acknowledge and value our differences while still attempting to move closer to a more considered and shared approach to mental health nursing knowledge.

Commentary 9.7
A Tale of Two Mental Health Nursing Traditions

Ian Norman

The chapters in this book set out visions of the past, present and future development of mental health nursing in the UK. In their diversity they capture the
coexistence of two traditions, which shape debate about the proper focus and
function of British mental health nursing today; I refer to these here as the
interpersonal relations and the evidence-based health care traditions. In this commentary I point to examples of these two traditions in this book and reflect on
their influence on mental health nurse education in my own institution, King's
College London.

The debate about the proper focus and function of mental health nursing has
been detailed elsewhere; see, for example, Tilley (1997) and Repper (2000). The
debate is between those nurses who are concerned primarily with understanding
the *process* of nursing as a discrete activity based on the *relationship* between the
nurse and individual *person* in *distress*, and those who are concerned primarily
with *interventions* or *treatments* for *patients* with diagnosed mental *illness*. Those
nurses in the former group draw primarily upon the interpersonal relations
tradition to support their case and those in the latter group on the evidence-
based health care tradition. In practice, most practising mental health nurses
occupy the middle ground between these extremes and draw upon both traditions to a varying extent in their work.

The interpersonal relations tradition has its origins in psychodynamic principles and owes much to the work of Hildegard Peplau, for whom nursing was
an important, therapeutic interpersonal process characterised by overlapping
and interlocking phases of the nurse–patient relationship. For Peplau the role of
counsellor or psychotherapist is at the heart of psychiatric nursing. Through the
medium of nurses' relationships with patients the aim of nursing is to create
conditions that promote health and promote the 'forward movement of personality in the direction of creative, constructive, productive, personal and community
living' (Peplau 1952). In contemporary mental health nursing the interpersonal
relations tradition is well illustrated by Barker's 'Tidal Model' (Barker 2001). The
'Tidal Model' holds that effective nursing occurs when 'the nurse and the person
are united (albeit temporarily) in a dance', when it is impossible 'to tell the
dancers from the dance'; a view that echoes Peplau's claim that 'it is the nurse
who is the agent of change rather than the mechanism or type of therapy' (Winship,

cited by Griffiths and Franks, Chapter 4). For Barker, 'nursing is something which involves caring with people, rather than for them or even just about them' (Barker 2001). These concerns of nurses in the interpersonal relations tradition seem far removed from the emphasis in the evidence-based health care tradition on establishing treatment effectiveness.

Several chapters in this book reflect the influence of the interpersonal relations tradition in mental health nursing. In Chapter 6, Forrest and Masters point out that users and carers involved in design and delivery of their pre-registration curriculum wanted nurses to 'care with' rather than 'care for' people, so implying partnership, shared responsibility in the caring process and an equal relationship between both parties. These authors argue that evidence-based health care, as currently constructed, devalues the status and experience of users and carers. The influence of the interpersonal relations tradition is clear too in Griffiths and Franks' account of the work of the Centre for Mental Health Nursing based at the Tavistock Clinic (Chapter 4), aimed at developing new models of mental health nursing by applying 'systemic thinking' and psychodynamic theory, as pioneered by Peplau over 50 years ago. A third example of the influence of the interpersonal relations tradition is Carson's account of the development of a syllabus for the education and training of registered mental health nurses in a college of higher education (Chapter 5), which describes a programme organised around the student's progression from being a 'knowledgeable observer' through being a 'supervised participant' to being 'therapeutically involved' with clients. Carson cites Wright's (1997) description of 'therapeutic involvement' as a process of mediating the challenges inherent in the nurse–client relationship, particularly those that emanate from the emotions of both nurse and patient. Being therapeutically involved is, according to Carson (Chapter 5, p. 92), a measure of the competence of an autonomous practitioner and a standard that all students are expected to reach.

The evidence-based health care tradition has a long history dating back, according to some authorities, to post-revolutionary Paris when physicians such as Pierre Louis rejected conventional wisdom that venesection cured cholera, and sought answers in systematic observation of patients (Rangachari 1997). However, the rise and rise of what is now called evidence-based health care can be traced to 1992, when a group led by Gordon Guyatt at McMaster University Medical School in Canada coined the term 'evidence-based medicine'. This term has spread around the world and 'medicine' has been replaced by 'health care' as health care professionals in addition to doctors have adopted its principles. The evidence-based health care tradition within mental health nursing reflects increasing confidence in empirically proven methods for treating mental illness, a critique of current nursing practices for not having empirically demonstrable benefits for patients, and a conviction that patients have the right to treatments of proven efficacy.

The influence of the evidence-based health care tradition is most marked in this book in Gournay's description (Chapter 2) of the development of teaching and research within the Institute of Psychiatry (the IOP). Gournay's account of the origins of mental health nursing within the IOP brings back many memories for me personally. In 1988 I was appointed to the Department of Nursing Studies at King's College London to replace Julia Brooking who, as Gournay points out, became the first academic lead nurse within the IOP and also Chief Nursing Officer for the Royal Bethlem and Maudsley Hospitals. This was a hugely demanding job with a combination of roles which were later uncoupled with the appointment of Bill Lemmer to succeed Brooking as Head of the Section of Psychiatric Nursing in the IOP and Ben Thomas (and later Hilary McCallion) to succeed her as Chief Nursing Officer. Gournay later succeeded Lemmer in the former role.

Meanwhile in 1988, I became – as Brooking had been before me – the only mental health nurse within a well-regarded department of *general* nursing, which had a strong empirical research tradition going back to 1977 when it was established under the leadership of Jack Hayward. This ethos culminated in the Department at King's becoming the first ever Nursing department to be given a '5' rating (the highest achieved by a nursing department at that time) in the UK research assessment exercise; this was in 1996 under the leadership of Jenifer Wilson-Barnett. In the late 1980s the term 'evidence-based health care' had yet to be coined, but undergraduate teaching in the Department was located firmly in an empirical research tradition. For example, I recall that nursing models (including Peplau's model) were barely touched on in the undergraduate nursing curriculum, since they were regarded as anecdotal and untested. In those years I worked closely with Susan Ritter, the first academic mental health nurse to be appointed to Brooking's new academic Section of Psychiatric Nursing, to deliver an education in mental health nursing to undergraduate general nursing students based upon well-established theories of mental disorder. Our approach to clinical supervision, for example, enabled students to understand the contribution of stress and genetic vulnerability to the development of mental disorder by getting students to chart their patients' life events and family trees (see Ritter *et al.* 1996).

In the intervening years there have been important developments for mental health nursing within King's College London. In 1995 Sue Ritter and I together with other colleagues established an undergraduate mental health nursing programme in the Department of Nursing Studies. This programme attracted around eight students each year and raised the number of mental health qualified nurses in the Department from one (me) to three (at different times, John Wells, Iain Ryrie and Sue Gurney). Meanwhile, as Gournay points out in Chapter 2 the basis for post-registration evidence-based nurse training (i.e. nurse therapy–cognitive behaviour therapy programme, ENB 650; and the Thorn programme) was well established at the IOP when he arrived in 1995. Other specialist evidence-based programmes (e.g. dual diagnosis, medication management, family interventions in schizophrenia, acute inpatient care, community forensic nursing) have been established subsequently.

The possibility of merging mental health nurse teaching in the Department of Nursing Studies and in the IOP was considered. However, as Gournay explains in Chapter 2, the mental health nurses at the IOP preferred to keep 'psychiatric nursing within a broad multidisciplinary group' (at the IOP) rather than have it join a 'nursing family' through amalgamation with the Department. This reflected Gournay's and others' belief 'that nursing activities should be part of an overall integrated approach rather than attempting to develop research and education and training as a primarily unidisciplinary activity'. And so it was that Gournay together with nurse colleagues at the IOP embarked on a series of randomised controlled trials in collaboration with psychiatrists and psychologists in particular, to establish the effectiveness of selected non-pharmacological interventions for patients and the effectiveness of evidence-based training programmes in changing nurses' practice.

Gournay is mistaken, in my view, to regard the King's College Nursing department as unidisciplinary. In fact the Department developed a social science basis for research and teaching; it was and continues to be recognised by the Economic and Social Research Council (ESRC) for training ESRC-sponsored graduate students. It was therefore multidisciplinary, rather than unidisciplinary in a nursing tradition, which would have entailed recognising nursing models, for example. In contrast, mental health nursing in the IOP developed an approach to teaching and research grounded primarily in medicine and medical sciences, rather than being multidisciplinary in a wider sense. Only relatively recently, particularly since incorporation of nursing within health services research at the IOP, has this medically-oriented base been expanded to incorporate the social sciences, particularly health economics. My own view and experience is that being located in a Nursing department does not prevent, nor has it prevented, collaboration across disciplines. However, it is also true that Gournay's decision to contribute to a programme of research and education within the IOP has made an important contribution to mental health care and has gone a long way to establishing the current dominance of the evidence-based health care tradition in UK mental health care policy.

In the late 1990s the scale of the mental health nursing teaching enterprise at King's changed when the Department of Nursing Studies merged with the Nightingale Institute (which had previously incorporated lecturers from nurse training schools in south-east London) to form the Florence Nightingale School of Nursing and Midwifery (FNSNM) at King's College London. With one stroke this merger also created two independent schools within King's College, both of which provide training and education for mental health nurses. One was the IOP, which provides multi-professional speciality post-registration/graduate courses for highly selected students. The other is the FNSNM, which provides pre-registration nurse education for pre-registration general nurses and around 80 mental health branch students each year, some post-registration training that aims to provide evidence-based skills for generic mental health nurses to use in their everyday practice, and a range of multi-professional post-graduate programmes.

In summary, the development of mental health nurse education shows that the IOP and the FNSNM at King's College London followed different routes towards a multidisciplinary evidence-based approach to teaching and research. In the IOP it is founded on an affiliation of nurses with psychiatric medicine and the medical sciences, whereas in the FNSNM it arose from close association of mental health with general nursing and an approach to research and teaching that draws primarily on social science disciplines.

In conclusion, the chapters in this book illustrate the influence of what I have referred to here as the interpersonal relations and evidence-based health care traditions on the development of mental health nursing as an academic and practice discipline in the UK. Whether these different traditions of mental health nursing care, both of which are represented in this book, can continue to co-exist is uncertain. In particular, can mental health nursing in the now-dominant evidence-based health care tradition – which emphasises external, empirically verified reality – accommodate the more subjective, personalised interpersonal approach to nursing care in the interpersonal relations tradition? Views differ. Gournay (2000) from his base in the IOP calls for mental health nursing to get in line with mainstream (evidence-based) psychiatric research and practice. In contrast, Barker (2000) asks mental health nurses to respect diversity and difference in their ranks in recognition that mental health service users need different sorts of services at different times. This line of argument is developed by Frese *et al.* (2001) who argue that persons who do not have the capacity to make decisions are indeed 'patients' who need tried and tested interventions within the evidence-based health care tradition. However, as they benefit from these treatments they become 'persons' who must be permitted a larger role in selecting treatments and services for themselves. For these people a close relationship with a nurse who supports them to make such decisions may be crucial to their recovery. Understanding the nurse's contribution to this recovery process requires systematic empirical investigation rather than recourse to models of nursing that are untested.

References

Barker, P. (2000) Commentaries and reflections on mental health nursing in the UK at the dawn of the new millennium: commentary 1. *Journal of Mental Health.* 9: 617–19.

Barker, P. (2001) *The Tidal Model.* http://www.tidalmodel.co.uk.

Frese, F.J., Stanley, J., Kress, K. & Vogel-Scibilia, S. (2001) Integrating evidence-based practices and the recovery model. *Psychiatric Services*, 52: 1462–8.

Gournay, K. (2000) Commentaries and reflections on mental health nursing in the UK at the dawn of the new millennium: commentary 2. *Journal of Mental Health*, 9: 621–3.

Peplau, H. (1952) *Interpersonal Relations in Nursing.* New York: G.P. Putman.

Rangachari, P.K. (1997) Evidence-based medicine: old French wine with a new Canadian label. *Journal of the Royal Society of Medicine*, 90: 280–284.

Repper, J. (2000) Adjusting the focus of mental health nursing: incorporating service users' experiences of recovery. *Journal of Mental Health*, 9 (6): 575–88.

Ritter, S., Norman, I.J., Rentoul, L. & Bodley, D.E. (1996) Clinical supervision in psychiatric and mental health nursing. *Journal of Clinical Nursing*, 5: 149–58.

Tilley, S. (ed.) (1997) *The Mental Health Nurse: Views of Practice and Education.* Edinburgh: Blackwell Science.

Chapter 10

International Perspectives on the State of Knowledge of Psychiatric and Mental Health Nursing in Britain

Commentary 10.1
Conflicting Knowledge/s: User Involvement in the Field of Knowledge

Kathryn Church

> In every field of human endeavor there is a continual process by which truths become reconstructed as people make history. (Carrol *et al.* 1992)

My response to the *Field of Knowledge* begins with Stephen Tilley's formulation of psychiatric and mental health nursing as a 'fragile tradition.' His attention to the embodiment of knowledge by particular people at particular moments in time and space illustrates a recent turn that some academics have made in the way we do social science. However, less abstractly, I am captivated by the urgency that permeates Steve's chapter. I share that feeling. Though we are literally an ocean apart, I too am confronted in my knowledge struggles with the 'discontinuities of volatile academic, institutional, professional, and policy environments.'

I come to this writing as an outsider: a sociologist rather than a psychiatric nurse; and someone largely unfamiliar with the curricula and practice of mental health nursing. I am situated in a Toronto university that has a different and much shorter history than the University of Edinburgh where Steve is located. Yet I am under pressure from the same sources: 'the demands of corporate accountability and the pressures to increase performance to secure funding.' As he rightly points out, whether here or there, 'Our ability to tell our own story is in jeopardy.' I view the conversation begun by this book as an important means to fight back.

The story that I most want to tell is about what contributors to the *Field of Knowledge* refer to as user involvement. The Canadian policy equivalent is consumer or (my preference) psychiatric survivor participation. I would argue that it is one of the most significant developments in the mental health field over the past two decades, with major implications for research and policy, professional training and practice. Yet – at least in Ontario – it has become largely peripheral, sidelined by non-consultative governments, funding cutbacks, and containment strategies such as assertive case management and community treatment orders.

A similar pattern is reflected within this book. Indeed, the degree to which user involvement is or is not part of the debate is one of the tensions of its construction. Differing definitions abound. For some contributors, the term means strengthening client narratives in the clinical context. For others, it means eliciting client experiences for purposes of research and/or including their opinions in government hearings. In any case, user involvement is typically taken up at the level of individual experience, one person at a time, and never quite free of a therapeutic overlay. Rarely in these pages do we catch a glimpse of it as a collective process, for example, as something that involves democratically organized, well-resourced groups that are accountable to their members. This individualization (and colonization) is what allows critics to undermine participants, especially identifiable leaders, as 'not representative.'

I carried out policy development and doctoral research on consumer/survivor participation in the late 1980s/early 1990s. Over time, I came to understand it as practices of participation and voice that challenge the knowledge forms currently dominating the health field. The authors who come close to this view in the *Field of Knowledge* are Forrest and Masters reporting on user involvement in curriculum design/delivery, and Chambers *et al.* discussing user access to nursing education. Here, finally, we are presented with the flesh and blood presence of psychiatric survivors in a different social relation, namely, as colleagues in research, and co-authors in the intimate act of writing. Here, finally, we read accounts of how the direct involvement of service users shifts and reorganizes power relations in ways that are unsettling to professionals.

Although some years have passed, I continue to feel the impact of my first plunge into user involvement and my consequent 'unsettlement.' What I learned from this experience (and *how* I learned) led me to spend a post-doctoral decade working on contract either directly to psychiatric survivor-run organizations or to university-funded projects that necessitated central involvement of these organizations. The decision to situate myself as a researcher outside the academy and the mental health system was a result – at least in part – of alliances with the psychiatric survivor movement. It was about politics. I foreground this experience because, in fundamental ways, it created a different way of seeing/knowing. This, in turn, organizes my reading of this book.

I understand that most contributors do not share this history. They write from the opposite end of the spectrum, from positions of disciplinary and systemic authority. Their eyes are turned towards the center with its interlocking systems of treatment and research rather than towards the periphery where I have spent my time. For the most part, they are professionals writing for professionals by invoking sophisticated discourses of care, science and management. Regardless of their specific focus, almost all write from power. Such would be the psychiatric survivor critique, at any rate, though perhaps somewhat delicately expressed. 'Who is this field of knowledge for?' they would ask. 'Whose interests does it serve?'

Once survivor voices enter the mix, I am convinced that we must begin to talk about intersecting and conflicting fields of different knowledge/s. Reading through this book, I was struck – as I have been forcibly in the past – by the fact that some of us have had to struggle with the implications of this shift more directly than others. How relatively easy it is to produce scientifically credible knowledge if user involvement remains a disembodied component of the mental health field. How relatively simple it can be, for example, to run the highest quality, gold standard, top level, world's leading nursing research department when your location buffers you from the delegitimated experiential, mostly tacit, often angry knowing of service users.

By contrast, how difficult it can be to reproduce (the same old) abstract, objectified knowledge when you sit directly across the table from survivor colleagues, when you get a gut-level feeling for what they are saying and begin to see their transgressive wisdom (their humour!) appear in your own work. How difficult it can be, for example, to write even a single publishable paragraph when you are confronted with peers who do not give a damn about tenure. 'Let me come to love my madness and you to love yours,' they say. 'Let us not live in fear of awesome majesty of the mind.' And you, as Chambers and her colleagues discovered, fall into silence and incomprehension for months.

This is an important experience: not knowing and then slowly, with others, beginning to invent new ways of talking, writing, working. It was one of the recurrent freedoms of my status as a freelancer. From a small office in the basement of my home, I could focus without conflict of interest on producing knowledge from the survivor standpoint that would not only strengthen survivors' contributions to systems reform but also enable the growth of independent survivor-run organizations. The best of this labour was done with a small group of leaders dubbed the In Your Face Learning Academy as we studied the contradictory practice of survivor community economic development. It included experiments with research methods, writing, and other forms of representation. In addition to academic articles, it yielded a series of plain-language documents, a video, and a full-length, broadcast-quality film entitled *Working Like Crazy*.

Other practitioners have engaged in similar experimentation. However, can the lessons we have derived be systematically taught as part of a credentialed programme? I think, for example, about how working with the survivor movement caused me to change the way I write: to write from 'I,' to write with emotion, and to favour narrative. These strategies are consistent with a testimonial form that I call 'first person political,' one that I watched survivors use repeatedly in public presentations before government committees. However, the decision to mirror that form in my academic work proved problematic. While this speech/writing form enlivens both arenas, because it is particular and subjective, it is not considered legitimate in either. Its use renders psychiatric survivors inaudible to policymakers on issues of mental health reform, and allied academics invisible to their peers as credible intellectuals.

So, there is academic resistance, not just to the substance of 'outsider knowledge' but to its forms as well. That noted, I cannot discount the importance of formal education. My own legacy includes a radical experiment in humanistic psychology undertaken at the University of Regina (Saskatchewan) in the 1970s, and the equally provocative socialist feminist scholarship that flourished in the sociology department at the Ontario Institute for Studies in Education (Toronto) in the 1980s. These two schools – marginal in different ways within the spectrum of Canadian universities – produced me as an intellectual. Pressing against the class and gender organization of my family, they changed my life. Yet, even as I recognize this, I know that interruptions in the process – and in the formation of an academic subjectivity – were as significant as the training itself.

Like a modern-day Penelope, much of what I knitted together in university was either seriously complicated or completely unravelled by what I learned hanging out in survivor-run sites. I was continually 'unlearning' as people who are insiders to psychiatric oppression collaborated with me on various projects. Bridging our differences took a long time – on both sides. It was difficult. There were breakdowns in the process between us and the context that surrounded us: places where pivotal relationships ended and others began, where focal issues suddenly shifted or were displaced by external forces, where major breakthroughs gave way to stubborn dead ends. Nothing in my formal training prepared me for the actual dynamic of doing and sustaining this work – and myself in it – over a long period of time. I had to learn that on my own, informally, and in that process psychiatric survivors were often my teachers.

What becomes apparent here is the hybrid nature of my own fragile tradition: a mental health practice that took root outside as well as inside institutions of higher education, that was nourished by the tensions between formal and informal teaching, and that bloomed in response not just to established curricula but also to the *in vivo* knowing of survivor activists. The implication of taking this history seriously – which this book demands that I do – is the need to prepare mental health nurses for a more diverse conceptualization and practice than is currently the case. Toward that end I want to make a case for curricula that would incorporate changes in four interrelated directions.

The primary shift would be *from an individual to a group focus* for intervention. Here I am thinking well beyond running support groups for patients/clients to the task of coming to know and work in alliance with the self-help groups that constitute the user movement. These groups have been around and active to one degree or another since the 1960s. Yet the existence of a relevant social movement and the question of how to engage with and build it in helpful ways does not appear within the *Field of Knowledge*.

Part of the difficulty lies with the second shift that interests me: *from professional/client to collegial interactions and relationships*. In becoming professionals, we are taught to relate as knowers: from inside the privilege granted by credentialled knowledge, positions within organizational hierarchies and the resources that come along with them. We relate through the categories by which psychiatric knowledge is currently organized. None of this helps if we are serious about user involvement. Can we yield authority and control? More provocatively, can we work under user instructions? How do we relate if we step out of categorical knowledge of a population and into a more direct, personal relationship? These are the tough questions. The dilemma for nurses is to both understand the tradition that underpins their work and deconstruct it for the sake of emergent, more democratic modes of practice.

What it comes down to – the third shift – is teaching *nurses to work politically as well as therapeutically.* I recognize that the *Field of Knowledge* favours the discourse of science over power and yet we know that the two are inextricably tied. The curricula that I desire begin from power/knowledge as a single formation, not just in the abstract but in the day-to-day workings of how things get done, and who gets what in the distribution of our collective resources. There are some stellar examples of nurses who exemplify this position. I am thinking here of prominent street nurses in Toronto who are tireless fighters against homelessness, and for adequate shelters/housing in the city. Their work touches hundreds of multiply labelled people. What they know, the ways in which they have transformed their traditional knowledge, needs to be described and systematically taught.

The fourth shift relates to the site of teaching and research. As professionals, we feel at home in clinics, hospitals, and universities. We regard these as proper spaces for the generation and application of knowledge. Some of the contributors to this book are infiltrating these environments with user presence, participation, and influence. I support their work. However, my preference, the stronger strategy, is *to prod professionals out of our comfort (power) zones and into environments that are user-controlled*. The very unfamiliarity of these spaces and the new kinds of relations that they generate are a strong impetus for fresh knowledge-making. In the process, as with all of these shifts, it is vitally important to find ways of identifying and working with the ruptures of knowledge that the practitioner will experience, and the unsettlements of identity that will inevitably occur.

Reference

Carrol, W.K., Harrison, D., Christiansen-Ruffman, L. & Currie, R.F. (1992) *Fragile Truths: 25 Years of Sociology and Anthropology in Canada*. Ottawa: Carlton University Press.

Commentary 10.2
Response from a Canadian Perspective

Ruth Gallop

This text contains several layers of thinking, reflecting and writing. Not only do the various authors write their views of the fields of knowledge in psychiatric and mental health nursing (PMHNing) from the perspective of their own particular institutions, but also they are asked to read other authors' contributions and comment on these alternative or even opposing perspectives. A third layer asks international authors to comment on the whole from their own experiential or educational perspectives. As the author of this commentary has been educated and socialized in nursing through a Canadian academic tradition, the challenge of making any meaningful comments is daunting.

In Canada, most nurses are educated in a generic program, with psychiatric/ mental health nursing forming a small part of that program. Specialization takes place at the graduate level or in certificate programs. After a period of practice, registered nurses can sit competency exams that provide certification in psychiatric/mental health nursing. Significantly, nurses in all areas of practice are expected to engage in therapeutic relationships with clients/service users. As a consequence, knowledge of psychosocial nursing and basic interpersonal theory is taught in the generic nursing programs and is not viewed as strictly belonging to the domain of psychiatric/mental health nursing. Hence psychiatric nursing in Canada (or at least Ontario where I practise) is specialist knowledge geared towards helping clients who are experiencing mental disorder or distress to manage their illness and recover their lives. The therapeutic relationship is viewed as a purposeful relationship in which the nurse uses him-/herself in the relationship to advance the well-being of the client. In order for the nurse to be effective in the PMH setting, specialized medical-pharmacological and psychiatric-specific knowledge is needed and taught in programs. All nursing education includes courses on understanding, evaluating and utilizing research in practice.

Overall, as I reviewed these chapters and the responses, I was struck by both similarities and differences. PMH nurses everywhere recognize the importance of relationships and struggle with whether the focus of nursing should be an art or science. For us, such either/or debates stultify nursing and I argue here for a thoughtful and rigorous integration of the two. In this book, Gournay sits at one pole, committed to science, evidence and a multidisciplinary research approach in order to define the role of nursing. At the other pole, authors such as Carson and Masters and Forrest seem somewhat skeptical of formal knowledge or therapeutic involvement, and seem to suggest that nurses need only be caring and respectful – decent people in fact – without recourse to a good grasp of the theory of relationships. I would hope these qualities of caring and respect would be a starting point for all professionals – but not a sufficient end. Knowledge in the service of the client has to be valued. The argument by Masters and Forrest for the blurring of boundaries between service users and professionals is highly contentious and for many service users neither desired nor helpful.

As I reviewed the chapters, I found evidence of the specialized knowledge/theory that PMH nurses need in the UK somewhat lacking. Instead I found some chapters more concerned with stating the beliefs/values of the institution vis à vis PMHNing rather than the knowledge needed to practise. Perhaps this is due to the stated aim of this text as 'an investigation of the sociology of knowledge in British PMHNing with particular focus on the institutionalization of knowledge in different academic sites'. For some authors such as Tilley, the historical contributions and influences of one particular powerful personality still haunt the halls of Edinburgh. At the other extreme, for Gournay, truth rests firmly in the evidence of the randomized controlled trial (RCT) and a close collegiality with other health disciplines. The humanistic tradition appears to permeate many of the chapters without identifying its theoretical foundations. One has to assume that the scholarly work of students includes foundational studies in the humanities and social sciences and that this knowledge underlies their humanistic stance. Explicit discussion of the specific social science and philosophical knowledge embedded in the chapters would have been helpful.

A reading of the commentaries illustrates that the perspectives of the commentaries remain consistent with the arguments in the original chapters. Chambers *et al.* remain reflective, and Griffiths and Franks, writing from a psychodynamic perspective, defend the importance of therapeutic involvement. Gournay, while reaffirming the positivist position, also suggests that the authors have much in common due to their desire for user involvement. However, I doubt that the other authors would find much in common with Gournay's rather removed notion of involvement.

As I have suggested, I am struck by the UK authors' largely atheoretical perspectives on the field of knowledge. Several espouse the need to be grounded in the 'experiential' knowledge of clients and to be respectful of their moral distress. Yet this knowledge is not overtly grounded in a particular scholarly tradition, but remains implicitly humanistic. Only Griffiths and Franks speak of psychodynamic theory as a possible explanatory model needing to be taught. The breadth and divergent understandings of psychoanalysis and psychodynamics are glossed over here. On the other hand, Carson argues that even therapeutic involvement is distancing and controlling, making us wonder after reading several chapters what a nurse is supposed to do? While I have no disagreement that nursing is concerned with an individual's response to mental distress, understanding/respecting that distress, as authors such as Chambers *et al.* argue, is necessary but not sufficient in my view. As clinicians we need to go beyond empathy to promote 'growth', 'recovery' and 'survival'. This requires a breadth of knowledge; knowledge arising from not only the medical sciences but also the social sciences and humanities. Gournay would have nurses acquire this knowledge through RCTs using tested measures and quantitative methods. He graciously allows qualitative research as an adjunct. While I have no argument with RCTs (the Cochrane reviews have made an extremely useful contribution), excellent research whether quantitative or qualitative can contribute. In North America, all major funding agencies fund nurses conducting qualitative research (not necessarily linked to a quantitative study) or quantitative research.

What I find startling is what is not there. These chapters are virtually silent regarding knowledge of the neurobiology of the brain as it pertains to the human condition. Even a person firmly wedded to the interpersonal/psychodynamic view needs this knowledge since all interactions are mediated by the brain and a person's brain can be profoundly affected by genetics and life events. This knowledge can help us make sense of our clients' responses and behaviours and become a basis for the direction our interventions will take.

As I have suggested, I find perplexing the authors' lack of accommodation after reading each other's contributions. There was no conversation – ironically, as I suggest above, Gournay gets closest to a conversation. Some authors such as Tilley attempt analysis, parsing out the voices into the two major camps. However, reconciliation or recognition of the need for all the voices working in the service of the user is lacking. Finally, it is clear that the PMH leaders in the UK value the relationship, want users involved in both education and research endeavours, and want nurses to be respectful of the distress of clients and learn from this distress.

Commentary 10.3
An Australian Perspective on the State of Knowledge of PMHNing in the UK

Mike Hazelton

In reading the chapters detailing the institutionalisation of knowledge about psychiatric and mental health nursing (PMHNing) in various teaching, practice and research settings in Britain, I was struck by many similarities to, and some important differences from, the situation in Australia. In what follows I will argue that in the rapid and extensive transformation of mental health care in countries such as Britain and Australia, PMHNing finds itself at a crossroad, facing both threats and opportunities. How we manage the pressures and possibilities associated with mental health reform and situate our disciplinary knowledge in relation to that of other stakeholders in the mental health field will be important considerations in shaping an agenda for the coming decades.

In recent decades mental health systems in many countries have been transformed, as governments have implemented policies to better coordinate and direct the development of services (Morrall & Hazelton 2004). While these policy initiatives reflect local conditions they also exhibit common concerns, including respect for human rights, commitment to service improvement and cost effectiveness, and reorganising mental health services to become part of mainstream health services. In his chapter commentary, Gournay outlines recent developments in mental health policy in England and suggests that similar developments are likely to follow in other parts of the UK. The recent setting up of the National Institute of Mental Health for England (NIMHE) is intended as a focus for the strategic and economic development of mental health services throughout England.

These reforms have a ring familiar to an Australian commentator. Indeed, they address concerns similar to those driving Australia's National Mental Health Strategy (NMHS): that mental health services should be comprehensive, responsive, strategically-focused and cost-effective (Australian Health Ministers 1992). In Australia the NMHS has been underway for more than a decade. In the initial years (1992–1997) the main focus was on improving services for those with disorders such as schizophrenia and bipolar disorder. In the period 1998–2003 greater emphasis was given to mental health promotion and prevention and building partnerships in service reform while still continuing to improve services. In the late 1990s in response to surveys indicating a high level of unmet need for mental health care (Andrews & Henderson 2000; Jablensky *et al.* 2000), the earlier focus on the long-term mentally ill was expanded to give greater emphasis to population health concerns. These studies demonstrated that for many people with mental illness, life continues to be characterised by severe disability, discrimination, social isolation, unemployment and poverty. Moreover, and despite almost a decade of reforms, there remained a serious lack of community-based rehabilitation services and of psychological and psychosocial interventions such as cognitive behaviour therapy and psycho-education (Jablensky *et al.* 2000).

The decade of the NMHS provides the backdrop for the consideration of the institutionalisation of PMHNing knowledge in Australia. All of the questions, concerns, tensions and contestations represented in the chapters by the UK contributors have their Australian equivalents:

- the quest to identify what is unique about PMHNing
- the shift to a collaborative approach to education, training and service delivery, involving consumers and carers in partnership with education and service providers (Hazelton & Clinton 2002);
- concerns and issues at the intersection of mental health care and human rights (Hazelton & Clinton 2003)
- the rise of the evidence-based health care movement; the future of the interpersonal relations tradition within PMHNing
- how best to approach mainstreaming and multidisciplinary approaches to education and training, research and service delivery.

What are different, however, are the ways in which these questions, concerns, tensions and contestations are played out within the cultural, governmental and operational conditions that prevail in Australia.

Australia's federal system of government involves power-sharing between the Commonwealth and State/Territory governments. Implementation of national policies such as the NMHS requires close cooperation between these two tiers of government, with the Commonwealth coordinating the response to major issues nationally and facilitating reform, and State and Territory governments funding and delivering services on the ground. However, this separation of powers often results in poor coordination and cooperation in areas such as health care and education. We can find examples of this in the failure of Australian health and higher education planners to coordinate workforce and university enrolment planning effectively in the face of a severe nursing shortage (Clinton 2001). Thus while agreement on policy directions may have been secured nationally, the implementation of these initiatives can be uneven and poorly-coordinated within and between State/Territory jurisdictions. In many instances, planners and managers from different but interconnected jurisdictions lack forums within which to coordinate their activities; this goes some way to explaining strategic deficiencies such as the 'lack of national infrastructure for planning the development of the mental health nursing workforce' (Clinton & Hazelton 2000: 101).

Another example of the difficulties of coordinating the activities of different jurisdictions is the development of professorial chairs in mental health nursing.

To date, chairs in mental health nursing have been established in six Australian universities located in three States (New South Wales, South Australia and Western Australia). In a number of cases the development of these positions has involved cooperation, including shared funding, between a university and an area health service. This implies the need for collaboration between the higher education and health sectors, including joint clarification of the strategic purpose, aims and responsibilities of the position. However, in a number of cases there has been no move to reappoint once a position has become vacant. This implies a concern that these senior PMHNing positions may not be achieving the expected outcomes, or that the sponsoring parties are unable to agree on basic considerations such as a secured funding base.

The discontinuities that result from these jurisdictional problems have serious implications for PMHNing at a time in which changes in both nurse education and health service delivery require the establishment and consolidation of what Tilley, in his chapter, refers to as 'senior scholarly practice'. The question of senior professional and academic leadership for PMHNing has been raised in a number of recent government-sponsored reports in Australia (Clinton 2001). However, the failure to secure professorial positions in PMHNing on an ongoing basis leaves the discipline under-represented at the senior levels and threatens the ongoing development and transmission of disciplinary knowledge. Tilley also refers to the 'fragile tradition' at Edinburgh, implying that the transmission of PMHNing scholarly practice in that university has often been down to one or two individuals keeping the field alive. While this sounds tenuous, there is nonetheless a discernable tradition and this has withstood generational change and continues to contribute to the professional preparation of a new generation of practitioners and research students. Comparing this with the Australian experience, we note the lack of such a tradition (fragile or otherwise). Indeed, in most cases the generation that took PMHNing into the universities in Australia is still in the workforce and there is as yet little evidence of intergenerational change or tradition-building. While some of our schools of nursing are strong in PMHNing, none has as yet attracted international attention in this area.

In case it might be imagined that the institutionalisation of PMHNing knowledge in Australia has largely been influenced by factors external to the discipline, I want now to address developments within PMHNing itself. In his chapter commentary, Gournay notes 'the gathering pace of the implementation of an evidence-based approach to health care, and particularly in the field of mental health', before going on to lament that 'much written by my colleagues seems to be done so without any consideration of more general policy developments that have occurred in [recent years]'. The implication seems that the recent mental health policy directions do not sit comfortably with many in PMHNing practice, teaching and research. This would be equally so in the Australian situation. There is no doubt that we have now entered the era of the randomised controlled trial, evidence-based clinical guidelines and systematic reviews and that many PMHN academics are not only ill-prepared for such developments, but also openly hostile to the intellectual tradition that stands behind them.

The debate between the interpersonal relations and evidence-based traditions in PMHNing as represented in the chapters of almost all of the UK contributors has certainly influenced teaching approaches and research directions taken in Australian nursing schools. Indeed, both Kevin Gournay and Philip Barker (among others) regularly visit Australia and contribute to nursing and health conferences in this region. At present it would be fair to say that at the undergraduate and postgraduate levels the content of Australian PMHNing courses reflects the influence of both traditions, although this may vary from one university to another. However, at the research higher-degree level, the selection of research questions and methods heavily reflects a preference for experiential and critical approaches, and much of this incorporates both implicit and explicit critique of medicine, science and patriarchy.

Perhaps similarly to Britain, the majority of practising mental health nurses in Australia would be familiar with and draw on aspects of both traditions, although it may be that the policy-driven emphasis on evidence-based health care is increasingly shaping practice preferences more in that direction. However, I believe there would be considerable sympathy among practising Australian mental health nurses (and some of their academic colleagues) with the point made by Griffiths and Franks in their chapter that a balance needs to be struck 'between sound evidence-based biologically and pharmaceutically informed practice and emotionally engaged practice'. Indeed, White (2003) recently made a similar point in relation to the debate over qualitative and quantitative research. The main distinction here should involve 'good' and 'bad' (rather than qualitative and quantitative) research; there is a need 'to raise the quality of *all* methodological styles, not merely as a vehicle for the chauvinistic promotion of one particular approach (or a single institution, or an individual, for that matter), especially when this is at the intentional cost of another (*sic*)' (White 2003: 94).

In his chapter commentary, Gournay points to the demise of what he calls 'pure mental health nursing research', and expresses a preference for nursing taking its place within a 'common agenda for all professions and users and carers'. The recent mental health policy directions require that the PMHNing field of knowledge be approached within a more generic and multidisciplinary field. Many, perhaps the majority of PMHNing scholars in Australia (and I suspect this is similar in the UK) will not feel comfortable with this new way of doing things; there is already widespread speculation over the future of PMHNing and the rise of the mental health worker. However, to elect to sit on the outside may very well result in the marginalisation or even the demise of PMHNing as a distinct field of knowledge. These issues, which are well represented in the preceding chapters, are also evident in Australia.

I have suggested above that in general the institutionalisation of PMHNing knowledge has been weak in many nursing schools in Australian universities. I want to go further and suggest that perhaps the most important site for the institutionalisation of PMHNing in this country is the Australian and New Zealand College of Mental Health Nurses (ANZCMHN). With its origins in the 1970s (in the antecedent Australian Congress of Mental Health Nurses), the

ANZCMHN now enjoys a level of influence beyond what might be expected of an organisation representing only about 12% of the profession. Among other things the ANZCMHN:

- Has developed standards of practice for PMHNing in Australia and New Zealand (these have been endorsed by nurse registration authorities throughout Australia)
- Publishes a monograph series covering important topics such as evidence-based health care, service outcome evaluation, mental health ethics and clinical supervision
- Convenes an annual international conference held in different locations within Australia and New Zealand
- Has recently introduced a Credential for Practice Program for mental health nurses
- Produces the peer-reviewed professional journal the *International Journal of Mental Health Nursing* (IJMHN).

The annual conference and the IJMHN, along with a variety of workshops, seminars, one-day conferences and other professional meetings conducted in numerous locations, often outside of capital cities, have played an important part in the institutionalisation of PMHNing knowledge in the Australasian region. Indeed, I would argue that as the only organisation spanning all jurisdictions in Australia the ANZCMHN provides not only a unique (trans-)national forum for PMHNing but also the national coordination so vital to influencing politicians and health and education planners.

References

Andrews, G. & Henderson, S. (2000) *Unmet Need in Psychiatry. Problems, Resources, Responses.* Cambridge: Cambridge University Press.

Australian Health Ministers (1992) *National Mental Health Policy.* Canberra: Australian Government Publishing Service.

Clinton, M. (2001) *Scoping Study of the Australian Mental Health Nursing Workforce 1999: Report from the Australian and New Zealand College of Mental Health Nurses to the Mental Health and Special Programs Branch of the Commonwealth Department of Health and Aged Care.* Canberra: Commonwealth Department of Health and Aged Care, Australian Government Publishing Service.

Clinton, M. & Hazelton, M. (2000) Scoping practice issues in the Australian mental health nursing workforce. *Australian and New Zealand Journal of Mental Health Nursing*, 9 (3): 100–109.

Hazelton, M. & Clinton, M. (2002) Mental health consumers or citizens with mental health problems and disorders? In: *Consuming Health: The Commodification of Health Care* (eds S. Henderson & A. Petersen), pp. 88–101. Oxford: Routledge.

Hazelton, M. & Clinton, M. (2004) Human rights, citizenship and mental health reform in Australia. In: *Mental Health Policy: Global Policies and Human Rights* (eds P. Morrall & M. Hazelton). London: Whurr.

Jablensky, A., McGrath, J., Hermann, H., *et al.* (2000) Psychotic episodes in urban areas: an overview of the study on low prevalence disorders. *Australian and New Zealand Journal of Psychiatry*, 34: 221–36.

Morrall, P. & Hazelton, M. (eds) (2004) *Mental Health Policy: Global Policies and Human Rights*. London: Whurr.

White, E. (2003) The struggle for methodological orthodoxy in nursing research: the case of mental health. *International Journal of Mental Health Nursing*, 12 (2): 92–8.

Commentary 10.4
The Field of Knowledge of Mental Health Nursing: A New Zealand Perspective

Anthony O'Brien and Madeleine Heron

In this brief chapter the authors respond to the contributions of British authors describing the field of knowledge of mental health nursing, and provide an account of mental health nursing in one New Zealand postgraduate programme. The British contributors have touched on issues that are reflected in our own experiences, and to some extent our response echoes concerns already expressed. It may, however, be of interest to readers to hear something of how these issues are played out in a different social context. New Zealand health policy has influenced the field of knowledge in mental health nursing, in particular by linking 'advanced practice' to population health gains, and by expanding the scope of nursing practice. Advanced practice has come to be identified with the nurse practitioner role, including prescribing. However, the concept has much wider application in developing the nursing role through critical reflection and inquiry, and is not always associated with a credentialled role such as nurse practitioner. In the current policy context, the traditional basis of mental health nursing knowledge in interpersonal relationships has required reinterpretation as policy developments have created new opportunities for realizing the goal of improved mental health.

The first author (O'Brian) is a nursing academic who has been involved in teaching postgraduate programmes since 1997. During that time the second author (Heron) has been involved as a consultant, teacher and advisor to the postgraduate programme for advanced practitioners at the University of Auckland. We briefly describe the advanced practice programme using Wilber's (1996) 'holon' model, relating the content and philosophy of the programme to the four quadrants of Wilber's model. We refer to chapters in the *Field of Knowledge* with a view to making connections between our own work and that of our British colleagues. Our analysis construes mental health nursing knowledge as socially constructed, and claims that current health policy supports the emergence of advanced practice as a dominant discourse within mental health nursing.

We do not claim that the programme, or the model of mental health nursing knowledge, is unique. Other institutions in New Zealand may well offer contrasting views of the field of knowledge, although each would need to acknowledge the common funding and policy framework and social context in which all programmes are embedded. Our account is one of a range of possible ways of organizing knowledge to meet the increasing need to prepare practitioners to provide consumer-focused mental health services and to achieve the national health strategy of more equitable health outcomes (Ministry of Health 2000a).

Advanced practice is a relatively new concept in mental health nursing in New Zealand, but one that has a considerable impact in organizing the field of knowledge of postgraduate education in mental health nursing. Within that field of knowledge, research, mental health policy, nursing theory, cultural aspirations and consumer knowledge are organized to reflect the aspirations of various groups with diverse interests. This means that educators are involved in organizing a range of knowledge, a process that inevitably involves value judgements about which areas of knowledge are included and excluded.

It is interesting to note in reading other chapters in the *Field of Knowledge* the different philosophical traditions that organize mental health nursing in the UK. The critical tradition of accounting for practice (Tilley), the psychodynamic tradition of the Tavistock Clinic (Griffiths and Franks), the interdisciplinary evidence-based tradition of the Institute of Psychiatry (Gournay) and the rising influence of consumer involvement (Forrest and Masters, and Chambers *et al.*) demonstrate the diversity of approaches to mental health nursing knowledge seen throughout the *Field of Knowledge*. A small country is necessarily going to exhibit less diversity between institutions, although the different traditions are, to some extent, played out within individual programmes such as the one we describe. Within the constraint of centralized control, there is an inevitable tension between the field of knowledge as it might be constructed by the profession and that prescribed by funding and monitoring bodies. Forrest and Masters note that clinical nursing is characterized by 'technological' and 'relational' schools of thought, the former emphasizing the nurses' role in diagnosis and treatment, the latter the more traditional interpersonal role of mental health nurses. They argue for a rapprochement between these trends. A similar rapprochement is sought by Griffiths and Franks in integrating the human qualities valued by consumers with the professional skills of nurses. The emergence of advanced practice as a component of health policy in New Zealand may be seen as consistent with aspects of the 'technological' trend, emphasizing, as it does, an expanded scope of practice, including prescribing. In this sense 'advanced practice' constitutes a structural constraint on mental health nursing knowledge. However, advanced practice represents only one stream of mental health nursing in New Zealand, and the profession has clearly identified 'relationships' as fundamental to mental health nursing, even as nurses assume advanced practice roles (Australian and New Zealand College of Mental Health Nurses 2002).

Since 1997, postgraduate advanced practice programmes in mental health nursing have been provided by a number of universities in New Zealand. These programmes were developed in response to a number of related concerns. The loss of specialty mental health focus in generic undergraduate nursing education (Prebble & McDonald 1997) was considered to be contributing to problems of recruitment and retention in mental health nursing (Ministry of Health 1996). At the same time, reports on mental health services consistently identified the need for nursing education to adequately prepare nurses for practice in mental health (e.g. Mason *et al.* 1996). Similar concerns have also been apparent in the UK as noted by Norman (Chapter 8). In New Zealand they converged to focus attention on mental health nursing education at both undergraduate and postgraduate levels.

Deinstitutionalization saw the closure of stand-alone hospitals by the late 1990s, and created the need for policy development to provide strategic direction in mental health (Ministry of Health 1994, 1997). Part of the strategic direction involves infrastructure, including the development of an appropriately trained mental health workforce. In addition, since 1997 the Mental Health Commission has promoted consumer focus and the use of a recovery model in mental health services (Mental Health Commission 1998, 2001). As nurses comprise the largest single group of mental health professionals, developments in the policy area are of crucial significance for mental health nurses.

There has been considerable change in the regulatory environment in nursing in New Zealand within the past five years. The 1998 Ministerial Taskforce on Nursing (MTON) (1998) highlighted barriers to the realization of the potential of nursing, and signalled the need for legislative and regulatory change if those barriers were to be overcome. Since that time the Ministry of Health has committed to a population-based health strategy (Ministry of Health 2000a) in which nurses in advanced practice roles are seen as crucial to achieving improvements in the health status of specific populations. Mental health policy has identified priority areas in both long-term and severe mental illness and in primary care (Ministry of Health 1997, 2002a). Similarly, Maori health has been identified as a priority area for health gain (Ministry of Health 2002b). These developments have implications for what we regard as necessary mental health nursing knowledge. The epidemiology of mental illness, the social determinants of population health status and the sociopolitical status of nursing, as well as the traditional area of interpersonal relationships, all assume importance within the field of mental health nursing knowledge.

New Zealand does not have a long tradition of postgraduate education in mental health nursing. Indeed, the development, in 1997, of specific postgraduate clinical programmes in mental health nursing can be viewed as both an historical and epistemological break, with the emphasis on the generic nature of nursing which was the practice of the time. This practice arose following the dissolution of the specialist hospital-based undergraduate programmes in psychiatric, psychopaedic, and general and obstetric nursing in the 1980s (O'Brien & Prebble 2000; Prebble 2001). There are thus no historical precedents for existing postgraduate programmes, and no epistemological traditions to enable a simple comparison with the evidence-based and interpersonal traditions discussed by British contributors such as Gournay, Tilley, Griffiths and Franks, and Carson. This may be a good thing. It certainly means that new programmes, while they cannot benefit directly from the richness of tradition, do not carry the weight of history.

The relationship between the indigenous Maori people and pakeha (non-Maori) New Zealanders, expressed in the 1840 Treaty of Waitangi, is a distinguishing characteristic of New Zealand society. This relationship received legal recognition in the form of the Treaty of Waitangi Act (1975); The Treaty being regarded by many as New Zealand's founding constitutional document (Williams 1990). A raft of official documents refers to the need for consultation between the Treaty partners. The Treaty relationship, often expressed as a form of biculturalism (Durie 2001), underpins all areas of public policy and governance in New Zealand, including health and education. Its importance to mental health nursing arises because of differences in the mental health status between Maori and pakeha, the articulation of Maori models of health, and policy commitment to equal health outcomes. The Treaty is the basis of a working model of power sharing between Maori and pakeha, based on the concept of 'cultural safety' (Ramsden 1993; O'Brien & Morrison-Ngatai 2003).

The advanced practice programme at the University of Auckland currently comprises four courses: Evidence Based Case Studies, Narrative Case Studies, Advanced Practice in Mental Health Nursing, and Social Context: Mental Health Nursing. Additional courses in assessment, legal and ethical issues, service delivery, cognitive interventions, research, pharmacology (including prescribing) and clinical practicums are available for students who continue to study following completion of the advanced practice programme. Students have the option of crediting their completed advanced practice programme towards a Masters degree in nursing. Completion of a Masters degree forms part of the criteria for endorsement as a nurse practitioner (Nursing Council of New Zealand 2002). The range of courses, perhaps evident in their titles, reflects many of the issues raised by British contributors and discussed in the responses to those chapters. In particular, both evidence-based and narrative approaches to mental health nursing are explored and are not seen as inimical to each other. It will be of interest to readers to know that both Kevin Gournay and Phil Barker have been visitors to the School over its short history, reflecting the perception that an academic department needs to benefit from a range of influences in its development.

Using Wilber's 'holon' model, the various influences on the programme are shown in Fig. 10.4.1. While a number of models could have been used as a framework of analysis, Wilber's model illustrates the place of both individual and collective functioning within the programme. The model recognizes the interpersonal tradition and the social context that shapes mental health and mental health nursing. The assignment of components of the programme to one quadrant or another is to some extent arbitrary. For example, social constructionist theory (Quadrant Three), while it bests fits with a notion of the collective 'we', by no means denies the social construction of health policy (Quadrant Four), or the dialogic nature of the 'individual' encountered in the personal stories of Quadrant One. Similarly, reflection on practice (Quadrant One) involves reflection on cultural identity and the social context as much as on 'individual' characteristics. On the other hand, the Diagnostic and Statistical Manual (DSM IV) (American Psychiatric Association 2000) lies appropriately within Quadrant Two, representing the part of the field of mental health nursing knowledge that attends to objectified data about individuals. This means that the DSM IV can be approached

	Interior (subjective)	Exterior (objective)

I N D I V I D U A L	Quadrant One
	
	I
	
	Narrative case studies
	Personal stories of mental distress/
	    recovery and care and treatment
	Reflexivity: nurses reflecting on
	    practice, clinical supervision
		Quadrant Two
		
		It
		
		Descriptive case studies
		Formal history, assessment, diagnosis,
		    plan of care/treatment
		DSM IV
		Observation, containment

C O L L E C T I V E	Quadrant Three
	
	We
	
	Social constructionist theory
	Traditions and culture of nursing
	Therapeutic relationship
	Consumer:educator dialogue
	New traditions (advanced practice)
	Treaty of Waitangi
	Maori, Pacific, Asian models of health
	Consumer culture, traditions and
	    analysis
		Quadrant Four
		
		It
		
		Outcome expectations of funding
		    and regulatory bodies
		Nursing standards, competencies
		Recovery-focused care
		Mental health policy
		Mental health law

Fig. 10.4.1 Wilber's (1996) matrix applied to the advanced practice mental health nursing programme at the University of Auckland, New Zealand.

as a resource that contributes to mental health nursing knowledge, but is circumscribed by other domains of knowledge. Wilber's model accommodates the different, sometimes competing, discourses from which mental health nursing draws its knowledge. The model has been used in New Zealand to develop an integrated approach to mental health outcomes that supports Maori understandings of mental health (Bridgman & Dyall 1998) and to examine recovery, teaching, literature searching, staff training, governance and treatment (Norris & Platz 2002).

Consumer involvement and a consumer focus in education are referred to in several chapters (Forrest & Masters; Chambers *et al.*; Norman). There are two senses in which consumer voice is important to the advanced practice programme. The first is in the presentation and representation of consumer issues in course content and teaching. This involves consumer teaching and academic involvement in marking, monitoring course development and consultation about course content and delivery. Shared classroom teaching sessions are an opportunity for dialogue between consumer and nurse teachers (shown in Quadrant Three of

Wilber's model), and exemplify this dialogue in action as ideas and perceptions are exchanged and debated between teachers who are consumers, teachers who are nurses and students. Consumer views inform the assessment and feedback on students' course work and provide a further opportunity for dialogue. The assessment process and discussion of students' written work introduces perceptions that arise from consumers' experience, and which are only indirectly accessible through literature and reflection on practice. As noted by Forrest and Masters, attending to consumers' voices raises issues of the relative validity of experiential and empirical knowledge.

As with the expanded scope of nursing practice, consumer voice is not only a philosophical commitment of the programme, but also forms part of mental health policy (Mental Health Commission 1998, 2001). The second sense in which consumer voice is important lies in the purpose of the programme within the wider social agenda of health care. New Zealand health policy recognizes the existence of social inequities in health outcomes, and the programme addresses consumer issues at a population as well as individual level. In two courses, Advanced Practice and Social Context, the social and political basis of health care is specifically examined, with particular emphasis on extending the contribution of nursing to improved population health outcomes. This emphasis coincides with recent policy and legislative changes that have created a formalized advanced practice role in the form of the Nurse Practitioner (Ministry of Health 2002c), and have enabled nurses to apply for prescribing authority within their scope of practice (Ministry of Health 2000b).

Several contributors (Griffiths and Franks, Gournay, Tilley, Norman) have commented on the place of mental health nursing within multidisciplinary academic departments; Tilley and Norman noting the vulnerability of mental health nursing within generic nursing departments. The programme described here began within a Department of Psychiatry, but moved to a School of Nursing when that School was established. The administrative location of the programme seems less important than the philosophical commitment of staff to working within either a nursing-specific or a multidisciplinary framework. The current philosophy of the School is strongly in favour of multidisciplinary relationships in teaching and research. At the same time the development of the discipline of nursing is seen as important, and the space within which this can occur as crucial.

Knowledge is both socially constructed and socially embedded. What we regard as the field of knowledge of mental health nursing will reflect the social context within which nursing takes place, and the impact of that context on the values of members of social and knowledge communities. Although the traditions of mental health nursing may be fragile, it might be argued that they have been lent some support through their institutionalization in pursuit of national policy objectives in New Zealand. Wilber's holon model enables the diverse influences and competing discourses of mental health nursing to be represented in a single framework, although such a representation perhaps implies a greater degree of consensus about the field of mental health nursing knowledge than actually exists.

The influence of advanced practice, as an expert discourse, on the wider field of mental health nursing knowledge is something that remains untested at this time. Advanced practice, especially when extended to nurse practitioner and prescribing roles, has the potential to become a dominant discourse at the expense of the established tradition of interpersonal relationships. Whether or not that occurs depends in large part on how nurses integrate advanced practice knowledge into their existing theoretical frameworks. The profession's competencies for advanced practice (Australian and New Zealand College of Mental Health Nurses 2002) indicate that relationships will continue to provide the basis of mental health nursing, including advanced practice roles.

Mental health nursing knowledge is currently shaped by the interpersonal traditions of the discipline as well as by global trends towards consumer involvement in mental health care and the need to demonstrate the effectiveness and acceptability of interventions at both an individual and population levels. Such international trends are given local expression in particular social contexts. In New Zealand, mental health nursing knowledge is shaped by our unique history and social context, most notably by the relationship between Maori and non-Maori expressed in the Treaty of Waitangi. Health policy aimed at maximizing the nursing contribution to population health gains, consumer-focused mental health services and the demands of funders to see these policies reflected in education programmes all influence what constitutes the field of knowledge of mental health nursing.

References

American Psychiatric Association (2000) *Diagnostic and Statistical Manual of Mental Disorders: DSM-IV-TR*, 4th edn. Washington, DC: American Psychiatric Association.

Australian and New Zealand College of Mental Health Nurses (2002) *Competencies for Advanced Practice*. Auckland: ANZCMHN.

Bridgman, G. & Dyall, L. (1998) *A framework for examining mental health outcomes*. Paper presented to the THEMHS 8th Annual Mental Health Services Conference, Wrest Point Hotel Casino, Hobart, Australia, 7–9 September.

Durie, M. (2001) *Mauri ora. The Dynamics of Maori Health*. Victoria, Australia: Oxford University Press.

Mason, K., Johnston, J. & Crowe, J. (1996) *Inquiry under section 47 of the Health and Disability Services Act (1993) in respect of certain mental health services. Report of the ministerial inquiry to the Minister of Health, Hon. Jenny Shipley*. Wellington: Ministry of Health.

Mental Health Commission (1998) *Blueprint for Mental Health Services in New Zealand. How Things Need to Be*. Wellington: Mental Health Commission.

Mental Health Commission (2001) *Recovery Competencies for New Zealand Mental Health Workers*. Wellington: Mental Health Commission.

Ministerial Taskforce on Nursing (1998) *Report of the Ministerial Taskforce on Nursing. Releasing the potential of nursing*. Wellington: Ministry of Health.

Ministry of Health (1994) *Looking Forward. Strategic Directions for the Mental Health Services*. Wellington: Ministry of Health.

Ministry of Health (1996) *Towards better mental health services. The report of the National Working Party on Mental Health Workforce Development*. Wellington: Ministry of Health.

Ministry of Health (1997) *Moving Forward. The National Mental Health Plan for More and Better Services*. Wellington: Ministry of Health.

Ministry of Health (2000a) *New Zealand Health Strategy*. Wellington: Ministry of Health.

Ministry of Health (2000b) *Proposed Regulations for Standing Orders. Consultation Document*. Wellington: Ministry of Health.

Ministry of Health (2002a) *Mental Health in Primary Care*. Wellington: Ministry of Health.

Ministry of Health (2002b) *Te Puawaitanga. Maori Mental Health National Strategic Framework*. Wellington: Ministry of Health.

Ministry of Health (2002c) *Nurse Practitioners in New Zealand*. Wellington: Ministry of Health.

Norris, H. & Platz, G. (2002) A house with four rooms. An integrated vision and an integrated practice. *Incite*, 2 (2): 12–22.

Nursing Council of New Zealand (2002) *Endorsement of Nurse Practitioners*. Wellington: Nursing Council of New Zealand.

O'Brien, A.J. & Morrison-Ngatai, E. (2003) Culture and psychiatric-mental health nursing: providing culturally safe care. In: *Textbook of Mental Health Nursing* (ed. P. Barker), pp. 532–539. London: Arnold.

O'Brien, T. & Prebble, K. (2000) Reclaiming mental health nursing. Kai Tiaki. *Nursing New Zealand*, 6 (10): 21.

Prebble, K. (2001) On the brink of change? Implications of the review of undergraduate education in New Zealand for mental health nursing. *Australian New Zealand Journal of Mental Health Nursing*, 10 (3): 136–44.

Prebble, K. & McDonald, B. (1997) Adaptation to the mental health setting: the lived experience of comprehensive nurse graduates. *Australian and New Zealand Journal of Mental Health Nursing*, 6 (1): 30–36.

Ramsden, I. (1993) Cultural safety in nursing education in Aotearoa (New Zealand). *Nursing Praxis in New Zealand*, 8 (3): 4–10.

Wilber, K. (1996) *A Brief History of Everything*. Boston: Shambhala.

Williams, D.V. (1990) The constitutional status of the Treaty of Waitangi: an historical perspective. *New Zealand Universities Law Review*, 14 (1): 9–36.

Commentary 10.5
A German Perspective on Paradigmatic Issues in Psychiatric Nursing[1]

Susanne Schoppman

Introduction

In this chapter the position of British mental health nursing – as described in Chapters 2–7 – will be commented upon from a German perspective. I have not commented on Chapter 8, as it seemed to serve a different purpose within the book, and was therefore outside the scope of my analysis. Nor have I commented on the further commentaries made by the authors of Chapters 2–7, as these seemed to re-state the arguments and positions made in the chapters themselves. Before proceeding with the commentary, it is necessary to give a short overview regarding the development of mental health nursing in Germany, in order to clarify the position from which the comments are made.

Since the *Psychiatrie-Enquete* in 1975[2] the psychiatric landscape in Germany has changed. Since then, psychiatry in the community has become the 'new program' (Dörner 2000). Community psychiatry strives to establish health care and treatment for people suffering from mental disorders near to their places of residence, to improve outpatient community treatment, and to close down big psychiatric hospitals. Consequently the number of psychiatric units at general hospitals has enormously increased; large-scale dehospitalisation programmes have been established for reintegrating people with lasting mental disorders; more day clinics and day centres have been opened, and numerous social psychiatric initiatives have been founded (Kohl 2001). These changes influenced the development of the role and function of the psychiatric nurse.

---

[1] 'Mental health nursing' would be a foreign concept in Germany, where the valid term is 'psychiatric nursing'.

[2] The 'Psychiatrie-Enquete' was the report of an expert commission which enquired formally into the condition of care in German psychiatric hospitals on behalf of the German federal parliament. The commission reported in 1975 that the conditions were awful and unacceptable. Therefore, recommendations were made which led to a radical change in mental health care in Germany.

Thus, post-basic education in psychiatric nursing[3] was established. Although regulation of this education varies in the different Federal States (Bundesländer), on average the course takes two years and contains theoretical and practical components. The need for further education results from the contents of basic general nursing education, where there are only a few theoretical and practical lessons in the area of mental health. The further post-basic nursing qualification in psychiatric nursing concentrates on the development of social competence, self-reflection, personality development, and knowledge regarding group processes (Arbeitsgemeinschaft der psychiatrischen Weiterbildungsstätten in der BRD 1997: 712).

Legislation passed in 1991 established measures for staffing levels for inpatient psychiatric care (which includes psychiatric nursing) and also detailed and extensive task descriptions, defined as the standard roles and responsibilities for inpatient psychiatric nursing. These standards differentiate general nursing tasks, specialised nursing tasks, and (indirectly) patient-related tasks. The standard tasks in the specialised nursing area are designed to support the therapeutic interventions of other professions, e.g. participation in group psychotherapy, maintenance, support and enhancement of everyday competencies of patients, and sustainment of social contacts.

For the first time there is now a valid description of the responsibilities and tasks of psychiatric nurses in the inpatient setting. This description also applies to multidisciplinary teamwork and combined care planning (therapy and nursing). For assessing individual patients' needs, various nursing models are used; the Roper/Logan and Tierney model is the most widely used model in nursing in Germany (Schoppmann & Schmitte 2000).

As numerous publications show (Schröck 1991; Meyer 1993; Bauer 1997), there is also a far-reaching agreement that facilitating the relationship with the patient is one of the main responsibilities of psychiatric nursing. This understanding is also valid for psychiatric nursing in related areas. These consist of institutions such as day centres, psychosocial contact and counselling services, and supervised housing for people with mental disorders, as well as community psychiatric nursing services. Similarly, the responsibilities of psychiatric nursing in these areas are to maintain and enhance patient competencies regarding relationships, assist medical treatment, and enhance and support patient competencies for daily living (Dondalski *et al.* 1999). In outpatient as well as in inpatient institutions the care is in most cases delivered by multidisciplinary teams. In publications describing the responsibilities and tasks of psychiatric nursing in community settings, the nurses' autonomy is emphasised compared with that in hospital-based psychiatric nursing (Wolff 1999). On the one hand this autonomy is seen as positive, but on the

---

[3] Basic nursing education in Germany is provided in schools of nursing, usually attached to hospitals. There are only three basic nursing education programmes in Germany: general adult nursing, sick children's nursing, and care for the elderly. The latter is regulated by the legislation of the federal states; the other two are regulated by federal legislation. All other nursing education programmes – such as psychiatric nursing – are post-basic programmes and are also regulated by further legislation of each of the 16 federal states.

other it can cause problems, when, for example, nurses in crisis situations have to make decisions on their own without feedback from others (Bonfigt 2000).

In the context of a larger research project for the Ministry of Health, a board of experts has developed recommendations for outpatient psychiatric care (Kauder 1998). The board introduced a person-centred model of care which suggests that all support and care must reach the person in his or her existing context of life. All care should be co-ordinated by an as-yet-unnamed therapeutic key worker. Individual care and support activities are to be performed by mental health specialists from various professions, in a multidisciplinary team working across institutional borders, with overall medical responsibility. As with the concept of multidisciplinary care in the inpatient psychiatric setting, the planning and delivery of community psychiatric care take place through teamwork, but under overall medical responsibility.

With the development of nursing in Germany into a graduate profession during the last 10–15 years, there are more and more studies undertaken from a nursing perspective. In psychiatric nursing the need for science-based nursing becomes more and more obvious. Schädle-Deininger (2000: 33) identifies the following as necessary areas of research for psychiatric nursing: studies about the effectiveness of nursing interventions; studies regarding the facilitation of milieu therapy and of therapeutic relationships; studies regarding violence and aggression. Up till now there has been little research in psychiatric nursing practice, and in the developing institutions of nursing science psychiatric nursing is under-represented.

As this short summary of psychiatry and psychiatric nursing demonstrates, there is far-reaching agreement in Germany regarding the role and responsibilities of nurses, who, apart from assisting in medical treatment, focus on helping to develop patients' everyday competencies and facilitating the relationship with the patient. In Germany the emphasis on implementing the contents of psychiatric nursing within this framework varies. It is frequently geared towards the medical ideology of a single institution, which can have a behavioural, psychoanalytical, social psychiatric, or biological orientation. An original nursing discussion about the underlying paradigms has not yet taken place to any great extent. This is probably related to the very slow development of nursing science. Nevertheless, German nurses in psychiatric nursing practice as well as research and other academic work are very interested in the theoretical basis.

Consideration of the chapters in Section 2

Seen against this background, the first thing that stands out in the previous chapters is the richness of the organisations and people who contemplate, develop, and advance psychiatric nursing, as well as the long tradition of the field. It is a great achievement of integration to have gathered these differing approaches in one book; especially under the perspective of 'care wars' (Tilley, as cited by Griffiths & Franks, Chapter 4, p. 75), which seems to connect seemingly differing and initially contrary concepts of psychiatric nursing.

On first view, the variously supported positions appear diametrically opposed and incompatible. There is on one side a biological–medical concept of psychiatric nursing which is based on a natural science tradition (Gournay, Chapter 2). On the other side, users' and relatives' experience-based knowledge seems to have more weight in psychiatric nursing (Chambers *et al.*, Chapter 7).

These differing positions raise a question for me: which knowledge – the objectifiable knowledge generated through natural-scientific, quantitative research methods or the highly subjective, experience-based users' knowledge – shall be used as a knowledge base for nursing? This question is closely connected with another one, namely, 'Who is the expert on an illness?'. Are therapists the experts, or the affected people? The answer to the latter question is then tightly woven into the understanding of disorders/diseases; in this case the understanding of mental disorders. From this perspective, the chapters in this book show a development in just this understanding of illness.

The natural science paradigm

This tradition is underpinned by the natural-science/biological understanding of diseases, as shown by the focus on research evaluating services and training programmes and various studies on medication management, described by Gournay in Chapter 2.

The knowledge generated within this tradition is of great importance to psychiatry and has led to changes in the perception of mental disorders as diseases, their demystification, and their gaining a status equal to that of physical diseases. Also, due to neurobiological knowledge, for instance of post-traumatic disorders, there are several methods of therapy based on eye movement desensitisation and reprocessing (EMDR) which help alleviate the suffering experienced by affected people (Hofmann *et al.* 1997). This knowledge base also contributes to a better understanding of some symptoms such as the loss of speech during dissociative episodes (van der Kolk 1997), and to development of adequate nursing interventions. In this concept of disease, nurses have the role of supporting medical treatment.

The social science paradigm

In Chapter 3 (by Tilley) the tradition of the Department of Nursing Studies at the University of Edinburgh is described with a focus on the shaping and passing on of these traditions through outstanding nursing personalities. In this description Annie Altschul holds a central position. She immigrated to the UK from Austria in 1938 and became a mental nurse[4]. She gathered experience in the therapeutic community with Maxwell Jones. Treatment within the therapeutic community is based on a social organisation, which takes advantage of the social environment

---

[4] This was the term under which she was registered to practice, and to which she held (Altschul 1997).

to initiate changes in the patients (Jones 1953). It concerns the influence of the therapeutic environment or the therapeutic milieu on people and their mental disorders. Parallel to the development of the therapeutic community in Scotland, Bruno Bettelheim established milieu therapy in America. Bettelheim, following a one-year internment in a concentration camp in Germany, went into exile in America in 1939. There he was head of the Orthogenic School at the University of Chicago, which provided a facility for treating 50 mentally ill children. His assumption, probably based on his own life experience, was:

> When an environment can have such a tremendous power to achieve changes in the deepest personality structures . . . then it had to be possible to create an environment, which would have an influence as powerful towards the good as the concentration camp had in the sense of deleting the personality. (Bettelheim & Karlin 1983: 112)

Both trends – that of the therapeutic community, as well as milieu therapy – have in common that people are seen as products of their environment, which can have a tremendous influence on their development. Through this the understanding of disease undergoes a change as it is extended by a social dimension. The social circumstances in the family and environment of the ill person are accepted as meaningful factors contributing to the development of mental disorders. Logically, within this concept of disease mental health nursing is based on an 'ideology of democracy, equality, and empowerment' (Chapter 3).

The psychoanalytical paradigm

In Chapter 4 (by Griffiths and Franks) the focus is on depth-psychological and psychoanalytical (included therein systemic) knowledge (p. 15). Here mental disorder is understood as an intra- and interpersonal relationship disorder, caused by experiences during the psychosocial development of the affected individual or family. Consequently, corresponding therapeutic approaches are based first on understanding the affected individuals and their development, and second on interpreting them to make unconscious aspects conscious and thereby available to experience and changeable. Here, facilitating of relationships, with particular attention to issues transference and counter-transference, is accorded great therapeutic relevance, as the means of corrective emotional experiences. Again, understanding of disease is extended. Now the social as well as the inner psychological development are seen as causative in mental disorders.

Consequently, the application of this concept of illness in mental health nursing means that nurses are responsible for facilitating a milieu and adopting a therapeutic attitude that supports and enhances patients' emotional maturation.

The humanistic paradigm

In Chapter 5 (by Carson), a nursing education curriculum is tested for its congruence with the ethical principles of nursing. Unlike the previous chapters, there is no defined model of disease underlying this. Instead, the author explicitly sets out from the minimum common agreement about mental health nursing, namely that nursing strives to alleviate suffering. This is derived from the ethical principles of helping. The curriculum that is tested includes, in what Carson calls the practical part, several levels of competence which students should acquire in the process of their training. The highest level of competence is to be a 'competent autonomous practitioner' which is synonymous with being 'therapeutically involved'. Here the author grounds his critique. On the basis of a definition from Wright he exposes this therapeutic involvement as a form of control of feelings and maintenance of distance between nurses and patients, which broadly excludes emotional knowledge. The author concludes that the impression is conveyed that mental disorders are a danger from which the nurses have to be protected. This means 'practising in an unprincipled way'. Therefore, the author suggests two alternatives to the therapeutic involvement: first, to enhance the integration of emotional knowledge (with the support of literature and philosophy in which emotional knowledge is developed and cultivated); and second, to integrate clients' narratives more fully into mental health nursing.

Surely, with the aid of other definitions of therapeutic relationships one could dispute aspects of Carson's argument, e.g. whether the conclusion that 'therapeutic involvement' excludes emotional knowledge is well-grounded. Nonetheless I would support the author in his view that therapeutic involvement presents a form of control. By using theoretical frameworks like that of psychoanalysis deductively in the treatment and nursing of mentally ill persons, these persons are pressed into an existing knowledge-form and thereby controlled. This means also that therapists are seen as the experts who have the theoretical knowledge and the practical experience in dealing with mental disorders. Carson's suggested alternative, to better integrate emotional knowledge by means of education and cultivation, also represents – precisely *because* of education and cultivation – a form of control. This form of control, however, is further away from medicine and more closely attached to the tradition of the humanities. This means that every person, ill or healthy, has the chance to become – within the context of the whole society – an expert in emotional knowledge him-/herself.

The second suggested alternative – to more fully integrate clients' narratives into mental health nursing – is also related to the tradition of interpretative phenomenology. In contrast to psychoanalysis, where the patient's narratives are also of great relevance, interpretative phenomenology is (from the perspective of nursing science) less interested in exploring the reality behind the narratives than in developing a deep understanding of the experience accessible to the other (Benner 1994). Therefore, the interpretation of narratives in this tradition is not a deductive one in an existing theoretical framework, but rather an understanding of the other's subjective reality. In this sense the sufferer is seen as the expert on his/her suffering.

Chapter 6 (by Forrest and Masters) discusses how mentally ill people and their relatives could be included in curriculum development. As can be seen in Table 6.1, the central component (as in Chapter 5) is that of valuing the personal knowledge, based on experience, of all persons involved. This leads to an understanding of mentally ill persons, their relatives, and the professional carers as experts. It leads also to a blurring of the formerly clear borders between them. This viewpoint is based upon the understanding that mental illness can affect all people, and the understanding that teachers and students can be expected to disclose their own painful experiences. Here it is important to explore experiences of suffering from the perspective of people who have experienced it.

The inclusion of persons with a mental illness and their relatives in the planning of the curriculum is described as a developmental project having several phases. The first phase is aimed at illuminating mentally ill persons' and their relatives' opinions about what knowledge, skills, and attitudes the mental health nurses should possess, and exploring strategies to include persons with mental illness and their relatives in the process of curriculum development. The second phase aims to evaluate the process of strategy development and to define appropriate strategies. This is a systematic process orientated to scientific rules and can be associated with qualitative research methods, which also stand in the tradition of the humanities.

The paradigm of the subjective individual case

Chapter 7 (by Chambers *et al.*) discusses the role and the importance of the person and his/her individual experience. The authors complain about the marginal status of this experiential knowledge in mental health nursing education. At the same time they underline the transformative power of this kind of knowledge, which can contribute to questioning and evaluation of the knowledge currently known and the existing way of generating such knowledge. They argue for giving the experiential, individual form of knowledge a central place in mental health nursing education on the grounds that this would help break the prioritisation of detection and treatment of symptoms, and lead to more understanding for mentally ill people; and thereby perhaps reduce stigmatisation and discrimination.

In taking this position the authors attribute great importance to the subjective single case in mental health nursing education. This emphasis on understanding the individual, subjective experience also means that the suffering person is understood as an expert on his/her own suffering. This knowledge, though, is limited in that it is knowledge about one case only, not generalisable to other individuals or ill persons, and therefore different from the knowledge described in the former chapters.

Conclusion

If one looks at these six chapters from the theoretical perspective in which they are seen as differing paradigms, they need not be in each other's way. Nor need

Natural Science	Social Science	Psychoanalysis	Humanities	Subjective Individual Case

Fig. 10.5.1 The continuum of knowledge.

they exclude each other, as might be the case in the above-mentioned 'care wars'. Instead they could be assigned to a continuum of knowledge, with the natural science paradigm at one end and the paradigm of the subjective individual case at the other. In between are placed social science, psychoanalysis, and the humanities (see Fig. 10.5.1).

Knowledge from the fields of natural science, social science, psychoanalysis, and the humanities is generated according to scientific rules. It is possible to discuss and argue about the validity and generalisability of a certain knowledge (see Gournay in Chapter 2). However, it is clear that knowledge generated in this way is always theoretical, textbook knowledge; whereas it is impossible to generalise knowledge from one subjective individual case.

The paradigms differ, however, in the degree to which they look upon a person (for instance, patients or families) as an object or a subject. This also decides who shall be seen as the expert on the disease, assuming that the expert is the one holding the required knowledge. Persons affected by mental disorders, and also their relatives and friends, are definitely the experts for themselves. Nobody else holds the same subjective knowledge based on experience.

By contrast, professional psychiatric nursing is characterised by living with the tension between theoretical, textbook knowledge and the understanding of the individual subjective case. If it embraced only theoretical, textbook knowledge, and nothing regarding the subjective individual case, it would contribute little to relief of individual suffering. If it held only knowledge regarding the understanding of one individual case, and no theoretical, textbook knowledge, it could therefore only care for just the one special ill person.

Therefore it seems sensible not to put the various forms of knowledge in a hierarchy, nor to see them in terms of an either/or option. They are what they are – in tension with each other as a criterion of professionalism!

Acknowledgements

The author wishes to thank Gernot Walter, Nurse Scientist and Psychiatric Nurse, for the translation of this paper into English, and Ruth Schröck, Professor of Nursing Science and Psychiatric Nurse, for her support and encouragement.

References

Altschul, A. (1997) A personal view of psychiatric nursing. In: *The Mental Health Nurse: Views of Practice and Education* (ed. S. Tilley), pp. 1–14. Oxford: Blackwell Science.

Arbeitsgemeinschaft der psychiatrischen Weiterbildungsstätten in der BRD (1997) Stellungnahme zur Rahmenordnung der fachbezogenen Weiterbildungen in den Pflegeberufen des deutschen Bildungsrates für Pflegeberufe. *Die Schwester/Der Pfleger*, 36 (9): 712–13.

Bauer, R. (1997) *Beziehungspflege*. Berlin: Ullstein Medical.

Benner, P. (1994) *Interpretive Phenomenology, Embodiment, Caring, and Ethics in Health and Illness*. London: Sage.

Bettelheim, B. & Karlin, D. (1983) *Liebe als Therapie*. München: Piper.

Bonfigt, A. (2000) Psychiatrische Pflegeambulanz Werneck: Aufgaben, Schwierigkeiten, Abrechnungsmodus und Voraussetzungen. *Psychiatrische Pflege Heute*, 6 (2): 65–73.

Dondalski, J., Schäfer, W., Seidenstricker-Loh, E. & Weigelt, B. (1999) Konzept der ambulanten psychiatrischen Pflege, Institutsambulanz Kassel, Psychiatrisches Krankenhaus Merxhausen. *Psychiatrische Pflege Heute*, 5 (3): 160–62.

Dörner, K. (2000) Reise in die Vergangenheit. Sternfahrt nach Bonn am 9 Oktober 1980. In: *Wegbeschreibungen. DENK-Schrift über Psychiatrisch-Pflegerisches HANDELN* (eds H. Schädle-Deininger, S. Wolff & G. Walter), pp. 150–57. Frankfurt am Main: Mabuse.

Hofmann, A., Ebner, F. & Rost, C. (1997) EMDR in der Therapie posttraumatischer Belastungsstörungen. *Fundamenta Psychiatrica*, 11: 74–8.

Jones, M. (1953) *The Therapeutic Community – A New Treatment Method in Psychiatry*. New York: Basic Books.

Kauder, V. (1998) *Personenzentrierte Hilfen in der psychiatrischen Versorgung. Kurzfassung des Berichtes zum Forschungsprojekt des Bundesministeriums für Gesundheit 'Personalbemessung im komplementären Bereich der psychiatrischen Versorgung'. Manual mit Behandlungs- und Rehabilitationsplänen. 2. Korrigierte und aktualisierte Aufl.* Bonn: Psychiatrie Psychosoziale Arbeitshilfen 11.

Kohl, F. (2001) Grundlinien der psychiatrischen Krankenhaus- und Institutionsgeschichte in Deutschland. Teil 2: Von der Begründung der Universitätskliniken zur Entwicklung der 'heutigen Versorgungslandschaft'. *Psychiatrische Pflege Heute*, 7 (1): 16–21.

Meyer, B. (1993) Psychiatrische Pflege und Pflegeforschung (1). Der psychiatrische Patient aus der pflegerischen Perspektive. *Die Schwester/Der Pfleger*, 32 (10): 864–7.

Schädle-Deininger, H. (2000) Psychiatrische Pflege im Kontext von Bildung und Bildungspolitik. In: *Wegbeschreibungen. DENK-Schrift über Psychiatrisch-Pflegerisches HANDELN* (eds H. Schädle-Deininger, S. Wolff & G. Walter), pp. 25–33. Frankfurt am Main: Mabuse.

Schoppmann, S. & Schmitte, H. (2000) Pflege bei psychischen Störungen. In: *Handbuch Pflegewissenschaft* (eds B. Rennen-Allhoff & D. Schaeffer), pp. 535–54. Weinheim und München: Juventa

Schröck, R. (1991) Das Beginnen und Beenden einer Beziehung. *Deutsche Zeitschrift für Krankenpflege*, 44 (8): 699–704.

Van der Kolk, B.A. (1997) The psychobiology of posttraumatic stress disorder. *Journal of Clinical Psychiatry*, Suppl. 9.

Wolff, S. (1999) 10 Vorteile der ambulanten Pflege gegenüber der stationären – ein Plädoyer. *Psychiatrische Pflege Heute*, 5 (1): 3–7.

Commentary 10.6
An American Commentary

Shirley A. Smoyak

I discussed my contribution to *Psychiatric and Mental Health Nursing: The Field of Knowledge* with Steve Tilley, expressing my reservation several times that I could not imagine who the audience or readers would be, or what the 'deliverable' would actually offer. That reservation still holds. For nurses outside of the UK or Europe, many of the allusions to the structure of the educational systems require that the reader understands the language, such as qualified, enrolled, pre-registration and carer. This is not the case; while the language is English, there is no consensus on the meaning of the words.

How educators are titled also is different. Faculty in the United States, who are in college or university settings, use 'professor' as a title, regardless of rank (assistant, associate, full, distinguished), while lecturer indicates a person who is a casual contributor to classroom teaching. In the settings being described in the book, lecturer is the common word for faculty. Arrangements between persons in charge of university teaching and those in charge of clinical settings also could be better described.

What is missing is a mission statement. What will be delivered to the readers? The rationale for including a very long chapter (Ian Norman) on past nursing models, in the light of present-day changes in how the British government dictates how the curriculum will be structured and delivered, is a puzzle. That chapter fails to address the current reality of nursing education, in its specialist and generalist dimensions. Further, changes in what curricular modifications are required by law seem to affect only schools in England. The UK is not really united educationally, since Scotland, Wales and Northern Ireland appear to march to other governmental drummers who dictate educational policy there.

For foreign readers, a short section on the similarities and differences in the UK countries would be valuable. Is there one license to practice, or four? Are advanced practice nurses licensed at another level? Is movement in job placements relatively easy to accomplish? Are the salary scales comparable? How many doctorally prepared nurses are there? Where are they and what do they do?

Is there a consensus on the utility of 'prescriptive privilege'? What are nurses required to know if they do prescribe medications? Which medications do nurses prescribe? How is that regulated? Is pharmacotherapy considered a part of the nurse's role?

Description of knowledge vs. who is best

Rather than finding an explanation of various approaches to knowledge for psychiatric nurses, the chapters instead deliver a somewhat scholarly version of 'Who is best?', or 'Who is the greatest of all?', labeled by Tilley, himself, as the 'care wars'. Further, the chapter by Kevin Gournay stands out awkwardly because it uses fiscal data to prove the point of who is best, while other authors use scholarly work as evidence of productivity or excellence.

There is no basis for comparing one curricular approach or program with another, or one institution with another, because the authors were given free rein to write whatever they chose, rather than following a guide or format which included specific topics or ideas. The degree to which information is presented thoroughly is also very variable. Allusions are made to persons who would not be known by people outside the UK.

While the focus is the field of knowledge in psychiatric nursing, the reader has no idea regarding where the tilling of this field takes place. Authors describe several university settings, and related clinical settings, but there is no chart or table showing all of the programs where such work goes on. We are left without knowing how many faculties there are, where they are located, what their highest level of education is, or how many students there are. There are statements about being new and having a few faculty, but no basic data about the student and faculty ranks. We also do not know what the selection process was that yielded this group of authors.

Several authors provide references for articles, which are noted as providing full explanations of a process of curriculum development or evaluation. Readers would find it difficult to access these because they are in journals not readily available around the world. It would have been nice to have these articles appear, reprinted, in an appendix.

Professional associations and journals

There is no mention of professional associations in which the psychiatric nursing faculty or clinical nurses hold membership. While government appears to be a very influential player in determining how education is delivered, the forming of consensus about education, practice and research matters usually rests with the relevant professional association. The fact that no mention was made of these organizations by any of the authors seems to be a very curious omission.

I have participated in various conferences and symposia sponsored by the Royal College of Nursing (RCN), and have shared my research at the Network for Psychiatric Nurse Researchers (NPNR). At these venues, there has been well-articulated presentation and discussion about the state of the art in psychiatric nursing. I am not sure whether to conclude that these bodies are not as relevant as they appear to be, to an outsider. Or whether their not being mentioned has another reason at the root.

While periodicals, journals, monographs and books appear in the references, there is no chart showing what the major sources are. What do students, faculty and clinicians read? How many major texts are in use at this time? Has anyone conducted a vote of any kind to determine the tiers or levels of excellence of the journals? Is there a 'book of the year' selected?

Applied vs. generic science

Several of the authors offered apologies for not having identified a body of knowledge or contributions to the field of nursing knowledge that was specific, unique or unmistakably 'nursing only'. I cannot understand why these apologies are offered, or why nurse leaders and educators continue to think that a specific 'nursing theory(ies)' or nursing body of knowledge needs to be identified, claimed or owned. Nursing is an *applied* science or art, not a generic science, such as chemistry, physics, sociology or psychology. *Applied* sciences necessarily use whatever bases of knowledge are needed in order to practise or do their work. I never hear physicians apologizing for not inventing new knowledge for medicine. They simply use what they need in order to practice. No one owns a theory. Once shared in print or online, it belongs to whoever wants to use it. There is no theory copyright law; the common understandings about citing the sources of ideas, of course, must be honored.

Psychology is another matter. The discipline of psychology creates and tests theories about how and why human beings do what they do, feel what they do, and so on. However, the profession of psychology is an applied science, and psychologists who are clinicians borrow from their discipline colleagues, as well as sociologists and anthropologists. Some even use systems theory (which is not a basic theory, but a theory about theories, in the von Bertalanffy style).

I think I know why there is this obsession with identifying nursing theory here in the United States. When the National League for Nursing Education began to accredit nursing programs in the 1950s, they invented the requirement that nursing curricula should have a 'unique body of knowledge'. Deans of Nursing and their faculty looked about and said, 'Oh, my – we don't have that! How can we find it?' And *voila* – there was Martha Rogers, writing about her 'theory of man', which was not generic to nursing, but adopted as though it were. Dr Rogers tried unsuccessfully to convince Deans of Nursing and nurse faculty that her work was not nursing theory, but to no avail. Then along came Callista Roy, Dorothea Orem and Imogine King, all offering their versions of nursing theory, which were willingly snatched up and adopted to satisfy the League's requirement. However, I have read nothing about the British government, which acts as a kind of accreditor, having such a requirement for basic nursing theory.

During the 1960s, when I was teaching a course at the Rutgers University College of Nursing entitled 'Building Theory', I would invite Martha Rogers and Hildegard E. Peplau to come to class as guests, in order for the graduate students to hear them discuss their approaches to theory building. Dr Rogers was a 'from the top down' or deductive type of thinker. She started with the big picture, or universal occurrences (energy, rhythm, light, waves) and applied these understandings to events 'down below' or matters of concern to clinicians. Dr Peplau was a 'from the bottom up' or inductive type of thinker. She started with the data at hand (what a nurse and patient said or did), and then generated ideas to explain what happened. Her concept of loneliness is a very good example of how she generated ideas from actual data. The women were fond of each other, and delighted in debating which of the two methods was better or more useful to nursing as a profession and to nurses in practice. The students not only learned two very different approaches to thinking and theorizing, but also learned that differences could be shared and respected.

Users and carers

Both Chapters 6 (Susanne Forrest and Hugh Masters) and 7 (Mary Chambers *et al.*) describe how users and carers were involved in addressing the need to have input in curriculum and program development from persons to whom nursing practice was applied. Both chapters clearly emphasize the need to focus on the attributes and human dimensions of the faculty and students, as well as the scientific content. These conclusions are sound, and apparently were derived without the benefit of randomized clinical trials (RCTs).

Proposed sequel to this book

As a follow-up to this book, I think that an international conference, to which all players are invited to discuss how knowledge is best built, would be a wonderful idea. In one common setting, there would be users, carers, users who are now faculty, faculty who were never users, researchers who never nursed patients directly, nurses who were never faculty, administrators, legislators, family members, clergy, and perhaps some representatives from psychiatry, social work and anthropology. The program would be designed to provide clear descriptions of what was and what is in the field of knowledge used by psychiatric nurses. The presenters would be required to follow a set of guidelines to assure that meaning was clear, that explication occurred, and that the 'deliverables' or take-home messages would inform current practitioners and administrators as well as potential students.

There would be tabletop or booth presentations for foreigners, who could take instant courses in English as spoken in each country, or short tutorials in how education is regulated in the UK.

In this age of technology, the conference could be telecast with an interactive component. There also could be instant electronic voting, so that consensus about theories, practices and so on could be generated instantly.

Chapter 11

Dance of Knowledge, Play of Power: Intellectual Conflict as Symptom of Policy Contradiction in the Field of Nursing Knowledge

Desmond P. Ryan

Introduction

I take the majority readership of this book to be nurses rather than sociologists. I therefore see as my task in this chapter, rather than academechanically[1] running some sociological numbers over the material presented by my fellow authors, to bring to it some usable insights. To be more precise, I see it as my task to bring such insights to the ensemble of the material: to the book rather than the chapters. My contribution could be assessed by asking: if one thinks about the other chapters in a sociologically-informed way, can one see more, can one see better – can one even see something other? To achieve this I take on myself the freedom to rework the material into perhaps disconcerting forms. The promise of any science is not just to overturn the view of the object but also to transform the viewing subject. Galileo's telescope directly gave us Jupiter's moons; but indirectly it gave us the Galileo[2] on whose shoulders we stand to look at the stars. So, paraphrasing Gödel – 'Nursing is not sufficient to make sense of nursing knowledge' – I shall go beyond the data to make my sense of the data, to see whether there is in these pages a whole that is more than – or other than – the sum of the parts.

The reader will guess that I was not selected for this task for my naive and inexperienced eye. I have worked on questions of professional education and training since 1969 (Italian social workers, Italian teachers, Scottish nurses, Cuban doctors), finding deep socio-institutional contextualisation to be my preferred intellectual strategy (Naples University 1970s, UK universities 1980s, English

---

[1] I introduce the concept of the 'acadamechanic' in Ryan (1997: 131).

[2] 'When we modify our judgements about anything, we make subsidiary use of certain new principles – which is to say, we dwell in them. Because of this circumstance we actually make existential changes in ourselves when we modify our judgements. For we literally dwell in different principles from the ones we have been at home in, and we thus change the character of our lives.' (Polanyi & Prosch 1975: 62)

Catholic Church 1990s), and utilising as my method my own variant of grounded theory (Glaser & Strauss 1967). Specifically on British nursing questions I have worked in some depth on two occasions. The first was a fieldwork-based evaluation of pre-registration nurse training of (non-university) Scottish nurses in the 1980s. The second was a qualitative (indeed, a grounded theory) review of the literature on the effectiveness of UK Community Psychiatric Nurses in the late 1990s (Ryan *et al.* 1998), one indirect consequence of which was a brief period working in a basic nurse training organisation in an educational development role. For most of the last 18 years I have had an academic attachment to the Scholarly Community Formerly Known As the Department of Nursing Studies, University of Edinburgh. I have therefore been privileged to think aloud with some of the most gifted and intellectually adventurous nurses there are, at any point of their careers from aged 18 to some in their 80s.

The relativiser thus relativised, to the task in hand. My strategy will be to situate nursing knowledge in its hierarchy of social being, to connect

- its day-to-day work with individuals
- to the socio-professional sources that condition that work
- to the socio-political shifts that condition the profession itself.

We need to make some connections here because nursing is at one and the same time an individual practice, a professional institution and a social function. This makes the field of nursing knowledge especially complex, both to work with as practitioner and to conceptualise as analyst. While I accept that the world is culturally constructed[3], in an advanced pluralistic society the cultures that do that constructing are partial, multiple and cross-cutting. Hence in what follows I can only offer insights and views, not a global interpretation. My thesis is that this book shows us the field of mental health nursing knowledge in the UK being subjected to destructive shear forces from the grinding tectonics of the three-level system of individuals, institutions and social functions. There is a whole larger than the sum of the parts: a professional discipline showing 'psychosomatic' symptoms of unresolved identity conflict in a stalled process of institutional maturation caused by the UK's failure to devise a coherent policy for mental health as a social function.

Level 1: power *in* the field of mental health nursing

Since the quality of nursing is assessed at the level of concrete nursing interactions between nurse and patient, one might expect the bulk of a book about

---

[3] 'There are only cultural constructions of reality, and these constructions are decisive in what is perceived, what is experienced, what is understood . . . Science is . . . a cultural system of a very special sort, but it is no less a part of culture.' (Schneider 1976: 204)

professional knowledge to be addressed to this level. My first surprise is that this is not so. To qualify that slightly, not directly so. The nurse–patient relationship is central to the discussion, but practical knowledge bearing on that relationship is not.

First, two significant exceptions, the ones that prove the rule. Griffiths and Franks explicitly discuss professional–technical approaches to the mentally ill patient. From the explicitness, however, we learn that the approach to patients taken by nurses in their institution (the Tavistock Clinic/Middlesex University) gives priority to a non-nursing form of knowledge: the psychodynamic approach. They see the value of this approach in its capacity to equip the nurse to stay on task in distressing circumstances.

> Nurses can feel overwhelmed in facing and experiencing the sheer level of pain, despair, distress and invariably anger that emotionally disturbed children and adults manifest. Even more distressing for the nurse can be his or her experience of the patient's destructive refusal to be helped . . . which confounds the nurse's desire to care. Many nurses without appropriate skills and support switch off from the issues addressed . . . retreat to a professional persona which involves managing the 'case', professional distance or following rigid interpretations of their role and task. (p. 67)

Since nursing has to take place in this maelstrom of destructive confusion, the first essential for managing mental illness is some way of making an alliance with the patient. Tavistock nurses seek to understand their patients in a way that is ambitiously deep, broad and long term:

> All patients have the right to be listened to and understood at as deep a level as possible. We believe that psychodynamic concepts have the capacity to facilitate this understanding. If a full understanding is to be achieved it is important to develop a collaborative understanding with the whole person, not merely a relationship with the presenting symptoms, difficulties or underlying pathology. (p. 68)

It is also a way with formidable theoretical commitments – the 'psychodynamic frame of reference' is a means to explore with the patient

> [through] a consideration of what might be being manifested/communicated unconsciously, by a registering of the patient's transference to the treatment setting, other patients, their relatives; and/or through the nurse's counter-transference to the patient (which may be experienced positively or negatively). (p. 68)

> . . . how previous experiences . . . may be impinging on their present relationships.

> This is a nursing use of transference and its corollary, countertransference [seven references given]. Nurses provide in this way a relational container (in Bion's (1970) sense) for psychological disturbance to be registered and empathised with. . . . This notion of psychological containment can be used in the service of systemic awareness, rather than

simply as rules of conduct, physical containment or defensive rituals [three references, including to Isabel Menzies' classic paper]. (p. 68)

This is a powerfully presented scheme for effective nursing within a larger therapeutic tradition maintained by an independent institution self-referentially constructed around an established tradition of knowledge – but a tradition whose 'external' character is signalled by the multiplication of authority-giving references when its esoteric theories become foregrounded. I present it at some length because this is what I was expecting to see more of in a book about the field of nursing knowledge: a conceptually articulated scheme of professionally applicable knowledge, theoretically framed, institutionally embodied, and practically warranted. Why therefore are the other chapters not more like this?

Evidence for a possible answer comes from the second paper presenting material related to practical knowledge bearing on the nurse–patient relationship, that by Ian Norman. We profit here from the historical overview developed by Norman for his English National Board study of the changing educational needs of nurses practising in different settings. Norman brings to our attention the sociological importance of the switch in emphasis to community care in the early 1980s, 'a time when the view that institutional psychiatric care was a thing of the past and community care its natural replacement went unchallenged' (p. 131). It was also a time of recruitment difficulties as the post-industrial UK economy expanded opportunities for both educational qualifications and female employment just as the shrinking cohorts of the post-1963 demographic downturn came into the labour market. Nurse educators started coming back from job fairs with tales of school-leavers who paused in front of the 'Careers in nursing' stand being dragged away by parents saying 'You can do better than that'. Thus the (*pace* Norman) Royal College of Nursing's (RCN's) attempt to raise nursing's status as a professional career through Project 2000 combined with the need to equip nurses with the skills needed for the more responsible, less custodial work in the community to pull mental health nursing education towards a more developed and specifically nursing knowledge content. This was symbolised by the new emphasis on the independent therapeutic potential of nurses (e.g. Peplau, nursing models).

Unlike the other authors, Norman is giving us an England-and-Wales-level picture, not a single institutional one. Hence although the models of education he so illuminatingly portrays are located *in* the field, they are effectively 'ideal types' (Parkin 1982: 30–36), abstractions which float free from any institutional linkage, hiding how they reinforce or challenge relations of power and control in other dimensions of nursing work. Hence the detailed discussion of the two main models ('specialist' and 'generalist') and their two variants ('pragmatic' and 'unity-of-nursing') remain somewhat tangential to the main theme of this book. Nonetheless, his consistent connecting of views for or against this or that approach to education and training to the wider context of social and political change makes his chapter of greater value to reflections on Level 3, the meta-field level. As this is where we grapple with the meta-question concerning the skewed approaches taken by a core of significant chapters, we shall come back to it.

Level 2: power *over* the field – when mental health knowledge is not nursing knowledge

We have several authors who, by the forcefulness with which they emphasise the *purpose* of knowledge in this field, can also help us answer the question why there are not more chapters that present theoretically framed applicable knowledge in its institutional embodiment. In the process of offering us competing ends for nursing knowledge they progress us towards such a question as: is there in fact a *field of nursing knowledge* here?

Competing ends for nursing knowledge are offered to us by, on the one hand, the chapters by Carson, by Forrest and Masters and by Chambers *et al.*, and, on the other hand, the chapter by Gournay. These chapters have in common (for this reader) a surprising conclusion: nurses are not the people who should (in the final analysis) determine what mental health nursing knowledge should be. The first group I read as saying it should be mental health service users, Gournay I read as saying it should be the psychiatrist-led mental health services research team.

Gournay's splendidly forthright and comprehensively referential paper is the fulcrum on which the collection turns; without it we would be really hard-pressed to know what the other authors were on about. In a more personally situated way than Norman, Gournay is the window up into the larger political–professional world by which UK nursing is constructed and reconstructed. Looking over his shoulder we see how the top power players exchange resources across boundaries which are impenetrable to players lower down. Research funders, hegemonic professionals like Sir David Goldberg, government/policy makers and institutional leaders are involved (and involve Gournay) in working relations across multi-sectoral networks. Gournay has secured entry into 'the Establishment' of UK mental health. He is fully reflexive in locating himself in both his institution and his intellectual genealogy as power systems. Sir David Goldberg has moved and shaken the Institute of Psychiatry – 'the world's leading research institution in mental health health' (p. 18) – in such a way that it is both more effective in delivering validated psychiatric services to the UK and more accommodating to a leadership role for Kevin Gournay[4]. Gournay's demonstrated capacity to deliver on the leadership role written for him has been recognised institutionally by the status of professor and socially with the honour of Commander of the British Empire. In his turn Gournay recognises the wisdom of the Goldbergian strategy for excellence in mental health services: scientifically valid research methods sifting purportedly therapeutic interventions to provide the

---

[4] 'Sir David ensured that others (including myself) were placed in real positions of influence on initiatives that included the reshaping of education and the foundation of various interdisciplinary research groups across the Institute. Sir David also encouraged all Health Services Research staff to develop and improve the Institute's relationship with the Government via its links with the Department of Health.' (p. 19)

mental health services with an effective and efficient set of knowledge resources with which to deliver clinical care to patients.

Not the least virtue of Gournay's paper is that he makes quite clear that he does not believe in developing mental health nursing as a unidisciplinary approach (p. 19) [5]. This had no place in the vision of Sir David Goldberg.

> [Sir David Goldberg's] vision has included each and every discipline playing its part in the development of an organisation that would, through research, yield new knowledge, and through its education strategies disseminate that new knowledge and the accompanying skills to the workforce. I believe that it is important to emphasise that the philosophy of those within the Institute who have a psychiatric nursing background is that psychiatric nursing knowledge should be seen as but one component of a wider body of knowledge shared by other disciplines. It is at the same time an area that can only develop within partnerships which include other professions, consumers, carers, and, indeed, the general public. (p. 19)

Another thing he makes clear is his endorsement of the medical view that mental health interventions generally lack adequate theoretical backing:

> At the present time, the only interventions in mental health care with a well-developed background theory are psychological interventions such as Cognitive Behavioural Therapy.[6] We obviously need to continue with our attempts to develop a theoretical understanding of what components of mental health nursing are effective. Simply put, it is our view that we should start almost with a tabula rasa and cast aside various archaic theories which continue to preoccupy many nursing academics and which are merely a source of frustration. (p. 28)

Nursing research has wasted too much time on 'endless explorations' of theory and not enough has been spent on 'operationalising the active components of interventions' [the analogy from the model of pharmaceutical effectiveness is adopted by Gournay from a Medical Research Council document on disseminating proven interventions (Chapter 2, p. 28)].

These excerpts from Gournay's work seem to me evidence that he has played a brilliant role promoting the power and influence of his institution, (his segment[7]

---

[5] In fact he seems hardly to believe in mental health nursing at all – he never uses the term for Institute of Psychiatry staff, preferring 'psychiatric nursing/nurses'. I take Gournay to be self-aware in this formulation, e.g. 'mental health nursing' exists outside the Institute, even among colleagues at their associated institution, King's College, London.

[6] Without wishing to embark on a sociology of individuals, it may be useful to relate Gournay's research training in psychology to the observation of Ben-David and Collins that when individuals trained in high-status disciplines accept posts in disciplines of lower rank, they may continue to adhere to the values of their former reference group and to apply its methods and practices in the new discipline, thereby generating a new paradigm (Ben-David & Collins 1966: 451).

[7] (Bucher & Strauss 1961).

of) his profession, and (his paradigm[8] within) his science. However, they also suggest to me that his framing of mental health nursing disciplinary knowledge verges on the reductive. Psychiatric nursing in the Institute may see itself as one component of a multidisciplinary research team, but Gournay frames it almost as a whole/part relation, where medicine constructs the whole within which nursing plays its subordinate part. Gournay speaks as one who 'leverages' massively more power than any other author, and clearly he helps his institution to do the same. However, within the context of this book it also looks as though he has lost control of the nursing business to a larger, better capitalised and more worldly wise operation. His successful alignment of nursing within the medical model may be a solution to the small, functional problem (knowledge for use by mental health services); but to the larger, societal problem (knowledge of mental health in society) his success may be problematic.

I say this from my reading of the other group of papers, particularly those by Forrest and Masters and by Chambers *et al.* Here again I have no space to do other than come straight to a sociological point. These authors agree that the knowledge that really matters is not nursing knowledge. Unlike Gournay and Goldberg, however, they believe the knowledge that matters is the experiential knowledge of users of mental health services.

Chambers *et al.* cleave the field of knowledge in two from the first line of text, a dedication to the memory of a 'survivor activist' whose contribution to the field of knowledge 'continues through those he inspired' – presumably at least one member of the writing team. In evidence-based medicine terms Pete Shaughnessy was, as a psychiatric service user and suicide, not a clinical success story, so it is paradoxical that he is publicly honoured as inspiring mental health professionals. However, there is more to come: another member of the writing team has an inspirational contribution from a user of mental health services with which he insists the team come to terms; but the author in this case is himself, and the team have reproduced his challenging textual behaviour to show what it was that stopped them in their authorial tracks for several months.

Less dramatically, Forrest and Masters make a similar case: that both the curriculum and treatments in mental health nursing are driven by external forces, and that this has resulted in a doubly dualistic model determining the experience of users: that there are 'caring with' and 'caring for' models in practice, and there are 'learning with' and 'learning about' models in education. The latter models objectify service users into diagnosed patients, making them less able to be befriended by nurses as 'helpers' on their journey through life and leading them to devalue effective therapeutic approaches of the kind disseminated to teachers by the Institute of Psychiatry and by externally driven curricula. The attempt to involve users in curriculum design was intended to escape this destructive vicious circle.

What is going on behind this reaching for new forms of knowledge? I offer as a conjectural answer that a Galileo-style paradigm shift is relativising professional

---

[8] (Kuhn 1970).

nursing knowledge before our very eyes. For these nurses, the patient has ceased to be the content of the picture, the view through the observation window, the details on the Kardex, the object of intervention, the theme of the expert analysis, but has become the vantage point from which to view, the subject of 'autovention', the author of the plan of care, the active agent of mentally ill wellbeing. When the sovereign perspective passes to the patient, the provider-driven approach based on validated technical knowledge turns out to be a stumbling block to a higher-order outcome, in this case the emergence of an inclusive society in which the mentally ill live lives of the highest quality feasible in their particular circumstances. From behind the elaborate socio-conceptual screens that constructed them as 'cases' (cf. Griffiths and Franks above) there metamorphose the persons-in-relation served by humanistic institutions so fundamental to one of the progenitors of Tilley's 'fragile tradition', John Macmurray (pp. 35–7). Objects become subjects.

This reminds us of the importance to our analysis of what purpose is attributed to nursing knowledge by each of our authors. Gournay does not speak of an inclusive society as part of Sir David's vision, nor was it the objective behind Institute nursing interventions or the driver of the research validating the knowledge needed to support the nursing function. Nor did Forrest and Masters and Chambers *et al.* have such a vision when they set out to write their chapters. However, it seems to me that such a vision was thrust upon them by the involvement of users/survivors, who dragged them from prioritising abstract principles to honouring lived experience and promoting the acquisition of personal meaning. Forrest and Masters emphasise the impact on them all of the process they went through together, involvement in which changed them personally as nurses/teachers, and fostered responses to the needs of users which brought them into new identities as 'also-patients'/'also-carers'. Subjects become 'double-subjects', amphibians at home both in the environment of scientific treatments and in personal distress.

Chambers *et al.* found that they could not actually progress the writing they were committed to until they had to some degree created an inclusive micro-society among themselves, one in which mental illness was a lived-with reality, not an objectified topic for teaching and research. This micro-society, too, provided a process-space for new identities.

> In the same way that user knowledge . . . challenges the validity and status of other previously taken-for-granted knowledge, these pieces of personal writing challenged the other authors to consider their positions, actions and approach more carefully. These pieces meant that we had to start communicating more openly and honestly if we were to be able to co-create something of value. They forced the issue. (Chapter 7, p. 122)

A similar confrontation with issues of identity emerges from reading the chapter by Alex Carson, who asks: where do you go if the principled review you conduct of the practice of your institution (Chapter 5, p. 86) suggests that your curriculum is more conducive to a technology of intervention/control than to an ethic of help? And if it suggests that nursing theory and 'Sherlock Holmes curricula' (narrowly rational and emotionally repressed) pre-construct patients in a reductive manner as foils to nurses' therapeutic involvement as bio-psycho-social agents? Carson's anxiety parallels the 'experientialists' group above, that nurses are being constructed as tools to amend the lives of the mentally ill. However, whereas the experientialists might wish to contest the *technical* instrumentalisation of nurses by (ultimately) scientific medicine, I see Carson as challenging their *moral* exploitation by (ultimately) society. Respect for persons as whole persons, for people's psychological integrity even when it is flawed, can be subordinated to therapeutic involvement as a non-negotiable professional programme. For Carson this is ethically unacceptable[9].

These four chapters on institutional approaches to nursing knowledge precipitate a more radical fracture in my interpretation than expected. The exemplarily scientific and institutionally successful approach presented by Gournay is seen as discrepant, at the face-to-face level, with honouring the integrity of the person of the patient, and, at the highest level, with the process whereby you achieve an inclusive society. One remedy is the involvement of users/survivors in designing curricula and authoring academic papers, which transforms those social processes from professional role performances to interpersonal engagement; and their products from technical-institutional items to political documents. Power is becoming very strange. For it appears that the power of nurses to construct patients as cases can be trumped by the power of patients to construct nurses as 'also-patients'. Case construction is overcome by communication, institutional roles are eroded by personal experience, therapeutic programmes are problematised by ethics, the ambitions of timeless science are overtaken by the imperatives of today's history.

Level 3: power *beyond* the field

To make sense one steps back, re-views. We see in progress an historic transition in the field of psychiatric and mental health nursing knowledge, a relativisation of professional knowledge which is undermining the autonomy of university nursing schools to determine their own knowledge on criteria internal to the discipline(s). I have suggested that this transition is contradictory, in that it has a single source (the political system) yet manifests in two dynamics (provider-driven science and user-driven experience) which drag nursing knowledge in irreconcilable directions. To resolve such contradictions requires one to reframe at a higher level of generality and pose a new question, such as 'How is it that

---

[9] A conclusion reached by eminent critics in the past, e.g. Szasz: 'To accept the existence of a class of phenomena called "mental diseases" . . . is the decisive step in the embracing of the mental health ethic. If we take the dictionary definition of [psychiatry] seriously, the study of a large part of human behaviour is subtly transferred from ethics to psychiatry.' (Szasz 1966: 86–7)

mental health nursing knowledge has come to be so determined by socio-political forces which are both external to the field and contradictory?'.

Kevin Gournay offers us a lead out of the impasse. In the first paragraph of his chapter he writes:

> Since the foundation of the Institute of Psychiatry in 1948, as a post-graduate medical school, clinical and academic activities of the Institute of Psychiatry and [the Royal Bethlem and Maudsley Hospitals] have been inextricably linked, and this linkage continues to the present day. Indeed, since 1948 the Institute of Psychiatry has provided the academic base for psychiatrists and clinical psychologists working in those hospitals. (Chapter 2, p. 17)

Is *this* perhaps the reason why Gournay's chapter is, by general admission in this book, so different from the others? Namely, that his institution, while putatively the leading research institution in the world in mental health research, is, to most intents and purposes, a hospital school? In other words, while all our other authors are working on the university side of the interface between professional knowledge and clinical practice, Gournay is not, but rather is speaking from the academic department of an asylum[10]? Further, that the power relationships to which he so obviously defers and from which he has so obviously benefited are those characteristic of big medicine[11], not of nursing, of clinical rather than of educational institutions?

Let us stick with this, indeed take it further by revisiting the historical background from Norman's chapter. He emphasises the transition (commonly referred to as the move to 'community care') from a system where services for the mentally ill were predominantly available through residential institutions to one where they are predominantly available in community settings. However, while considerable numbers of mental health nurses have 'followed the patients' out of the asylums into the community, relatively few psychiatrists have. Residential mental hospitals have remained the power base of the psychiatry wing of the medical profession, and the 1990s saw something of a power struggle between psychiatrists and GPs for the control of community-based nurses (Samson 1995;

---

[10] I use this archaic term designedly to expand the conceptual repertoire informing our discussion. We perhaps tend to forget how relatively brief (+/− 60 years) was the hegemony over the mental health system of the idea of 'hospital', between displacing 'asylum' and being relegated by the vision of 'community': 'The *Report of the Royal Commissioners on the Care and Control of the Feeble Minded* (1908) . . . signifies the official point at which the protective and segregative goals of asylum care began to be replaced by the goals of medical treatment. From 1908 onwards . . . the concept of asylum – understood as a place of retreat – was subordinated to the concept of hospital as a place for medical intervention.' (Prior 1993: 145)

[11] Gournay stands out in the group, as Shirley Smoyak notes (Chapter 10.6, p. 213), for referring to money as evidence of the quality of his group's academic programmes. While in British medicine such 'pound-scoring' tallies are accepted as proxy scientific discriminators between knowledge teams, this is (as yet) less the case in nursing academic culture.

Corney 1996), the GPs arguing that since so much mental ill-health was treated in the community, that is where the resources ought to be too[12]. Gournay has long been critical of the standard of mental health services in the community[13], thus it is no surprise that he should be found standing with the psychiatric team in this particular power game.

Now, a synthetic move from story to structure. In systems theory terms, the expansion of community care is an historical–functional transition but *not* a metasystem transition (Turchin 1981): we do not have the emergence of a new, governing level, but rather the establishment of two functions at one level with such inadequate provision for their co-ordination that conflict has become endemic at the level of knowledge-for-use. In view of the contradictory coexistence of residential hospitals and community care, it is reasonable to describe the field within which nursing has to make its way as a metathetelic monster (Wigglesworth 1968: 111), functionally enlarged but not morphologically developed, frozen in mid-metamorphosis with characteristics of both 'stages'. One sociological feature of this clinical regime is that it is dual purpose: it works at one and the same time to preserve the determining power of medicine over the clinical functioning of the system, but also to 'deliver services' predicated on the (qualified) right of the citizen-patient to determine his or her own care. Thus one part of this dualistic system objectifies severely mentally ill patients through natural science-style diagnoses and treats them with clinically validated interventions (often administered in custodial settings) under the medical superintendence of psychiatrists; the other part seeks to maintain the personhood of patients, to facilitate the enjoyment of their citizenship rights in the most normal lives possible through relationship-based support structures centred on devolved clinical management regimes. Ideal-typically, one could say, the hospital diagnoses a patient with a disease for which the best hope of a cure is rigorous science, whereas the community gives space to a user on a (possibly life-long) journey of 'recovery' (Deegan 1996) for which his or her best hope of support is responsive relationships.

The source of the tension here, it seems to me, is not that it is in principle impossible to integrate both these approaches intellectually – the New Zealand approach based on the Wilber holon model cited by O'Brien and Heron appears to have done so. It is rather that each approach has inherent in it a construction of the patient/user, and thus, reciprocally, a construction of the nurse. It is their self-identities that play the key role in prompting them to lean towards one or other mode of practice, and thus to one or other mode of knowing. It is also their

---

[12] Michael Shepherd claimed that '... acknowledging the fact that *the bulk of mental illness in any community never comes to the attention of a psychiatric specialist* ... brings a radically different perspective to community psychiatry, one which employs a socio-medical approach within a public health framework. Teamwork becomes indispensable, and the general practitioner's activities extend to close collaboration with non-medical colleagues, especially social workers, nurses and psychologists. And by the same token *the role of the psychiatrist is diminished.*' (Shepherd 1993) [emphases in original]
[13] E.g. (Gournay & Brooking 1993).

identities that raise the stakes in debate and make dialogue difficult and accommodation resisted, as the overseas authors have noted. Seeing *from within* one perspective means they automatically reduce the other: they look at each other through reversed telescopes: whereas relationship-based approaches have for some time[14] been seen in the psychiatric system as clinically insignificant (Gournay's 'archaic theories . . . merely a source of frustration'), scientific approaches are seen by community-based users as a necessary evil, strategically managed by the experienced among them to maximise the good things in their 'persons-not-patients' lives[15] (Shepherd *et al.* 1995).

The major contrast among the institutional chapters, therefore, is between chapters with a theoretical and clinical base which both constructs and positions the patients (the Institute of Psychiatry and the Tavistock/Middlesex) and those that are, in different ways and to different degrees, constructed by/in the interests of users/survivors (Forrest and Masters, Chambers *et al.*, Carson). My 'to different degrees' qualifier is an important one: it is hard not to read Forrest and Masters as having ended up in a minority space among their colleagues (e.g. being seen as a 'cult'). This may suggest something very important, that responding to users is one thing, but meeting service requirements is another. Users may break in to a curriculum-design process via working partnerships with sympathetic teachers, but there seems little evidence that they have much influence over the determination of UK service delivery as at present construed – even progressive Ontario survivor participation 'has become largely peripheral, sidelined by non-consultative governments, funding cutbacks, and containment strategies . . .' (Church, Chapter 10.1, p. 181).[16]

The contrasts between the two major approaches show up in a variety of modes. In epistemological terms there is a tension between science and experience as the primary authority. In knowledge terms, there is a possible reversal between esoteric and exoteric knowledge as the foundation for practice. In practice terms there is a differentiation between applying best science (theory +

---

[14] In the days before the technologisation of psychiatric care through the control of behaviour, relationship-based approaches had proven successful in such diverse contexts as Geel, Belgium (Roosens 1979), administrative therapy (Clark 1964), and the therapeutic community (Rapaport 1960).
[15] The dilemmas of transferring rigorous scientific insights to messy real-world settings (aka 'evidence-based practice') have occupied leading minds for a long time – cf.: 'I say moreover that you make a great, a very great mistake, if you think that psychology, being the science of the mind's laws, is something from which you can deduce definite programmes and schemes and methods of instruction, for immediate schoolroom use. Psychology is a science, and teaching is an art, and sciences never generate arts directly out of themselves. An intermediary inventive mind must make the application, by using its originality.' (James 1907: 7–8) Even mathematics gets transformed in real-world settings: '. . . situational specificity of arithmetic practice comes about because there are integral relations between activities like grocery shopping and settings like the supermarket.' (Lave 1986). Cf. Bowers (1992) on the situational specificity of mental health nursing practice in the patient's home.
[16] Note also that drawing the contrast in terms of the presence or absence of a positioning theoretical–clinical base leaves Griffiths and Franks on a different side of the equation to where they would be if one were to draw the contrast in terms of the nature of their knowledge, as several authors do.

evidence) to 'patients and responding to the needs of users. In identity terms the contrast is very significant indeed, most clearly signalled to us by Pete Shaughnessy's culture-shift in setting up *Mad Pride* (Chambers *et al.*, Chapter 7, p. 114): that it is no less reasonable that users should seek to assimilate nurses to their minority life-world than that nurses should try to maintain users in the majority life-world. As the old institutional order breaks down and the former asylum residents (patients *and* nurses) break out, the conceptual order breaks up and becomes a knowledge space inviting the newly empowered users to break in – not such a hard task now that there are acknowledged users 'on the inside'. There is a dynamically dialectical congruence between institution and discipline; change in one dimension is quickly followed by change in the other, which then reacts back upon the first. Sociological transition/fracture results in epistemological crisis (MacIntyre 1989).

In view of this, I am not surprised that, as Gallop points out, there is no 'conversation', no 'accommodation after reading each others' contributions', that the authors talk past each other, reiterating already well-rehearsed views rather than engaging with the alternative discourse. Schoppmann too feels that the aim of the book was intended to be 'integration of different viewpoints' and is disappointed by the failure of the authors to come into a dialogue together to achieve this. It is also not too surprising that, again in Gallop's terms, the 'breadth of knowledge, knowledge arising from not only the medical sciences but also the social sciences and humanities required to promote "growth", "recovery" and "survival"' is not reviewed (Chapter 10.2, pp. 187–8). One has to presume that much of this knowledge is made available to learners in all the UK institutions represented here, as I know it is in Tilley's department. However, I interpret these authors as leaving dialogue behind, so to speak, when they move from the level of efficient cause to final cause, to asking 'which knowledge for what purpose?' Not so much 'What are we doing in our institution?' (effectively Tilley's question to contributors) but rather 'What are we trying to achieve?' This seems to me to be psychologically reasonable: strong goals are needed to resist the unresolvable tensions transmitted into their life-worlds by the shear forces pulling the different levels/sectors of the mental health services in different directions. Under conditions of confusion and conflict, making clear 'Where am I trying to get to?' is sensible enough. However, answers to the question are more likely to be determined by values and identity than by discipline and methods.

I have interpreted the major contrast in the accounts as evidence that different parts of psychiatric/mental health nursing in the UK are actually coming from different places and trying to do different things. Of course they are not mutually exclusive: Gournay no more wishes to ignore users' wishes than 'the experientialists' wish to throw out quantitative research and proven clinical methods. However, I cannot doubt that their knowledge/scientific loyalties are to different paradigms, which I believe to be whether esoteric knowledge takes priority over exoteric or the reverse. In the dance of care, who leads – the professional or the user? Who is the 'expert' in mental illness, the one who has most knowledge *about* it or the one who has most knowledge *of* it? I believe this paradigm ambiguity has resulted from the intellectually shallow way in which community care and the acute hospital were juxtaposed with insufficient in-depth working out of how they were to relate to each other as different aspects of the life-world of mentally ill people. The policy thinking fell short of the political acting and left a conceptual mess which patients and practitioners have still to muddle through.

I am supported in this general point about the importance of structural arrangements by an analogous argument by Mike Hazelton. He points out that many of the unresolved tensions affecting mental health nursing practice and education in the UK also exist in Australia, but the dualism (constitutional rather than metathetelic) which he identifies as largely contributory to them is not that between asylum/psychiatry and community/users but between Commonwealth and State/Territory governments. I see it as significant that these governments' failure to create an assured institutional platform for mental health nursing has prompted a leadership group within the profession to set up an organisation (the Australian and New Zealand College of Mental Health Nurses) for the 'assertive management' of the field itself, including the politicians. Could this be the control and co-ordination centre that metasystem transitions need if they are to be successful at integrating disparate functions into a unitary system? It would be interesting to compare this radical evolutionary break in Australia with the conceptually more one-sided Institute of Psychiatry in the UK as contenders for the future hegemonic management of mental health knowledge. A propos national differences, I think it is also significant that in Germany, a country where mental health nursing science/knowledge is developing more slowly than in the English-speaking countries, '[a]n original nursing discussion about the underlying paradigms has not yet taken place to any great extent' (Schoppmann, Chapter 10.4, p. 4). For obvious historical reasons, Germany moves more slowly in re-engineering its institutions to secure political pay-offs through satisfying discrete interest groups than we have become used to in the UK. One may, however, take pause slightly before Susanne Schoppmann's verdict (p. 205) that it 'is a great achievement of integration to have gathered [the] differing approaches in one book . . . under the perspective of "care wars" '!

Conclusion

However, what if she is right, that this book is indeed a great achievement of integration? How might it be so? Let us leave the UK for a while and move to a fourth level in the hierarchy of social being, the overseas world. To focus our search, let us take with us some core sociological insights.

Before leaving we need to ask what it is that keeps in being our metathetelic monster, our dualistic mental health system torn between science and experience? Berger and Luckmann might suggest that, through the very debates and discussions we have seen in this book, this dualistic world has become to us an objective reality, our taken-for-granted objective universe.

The basic form of social objectivation is language ... [the] edifice of semantic fields, categories and norms which structures the subjective perceptions of reality into a meaningful, cohesive and 'objective' universe. This universe, 'reality as seen' in a culture, is taken for granted in any particular society or collectivity. For the members of a society it constitutes the 'natural' way of interpreting, remembering and communicating individual experience. In this sense it is internal to the individual, as his way of experiencing the world. At the same time it is external to him as that universe in which he and his fellow-men exist and act. (Berger & Luckmann 1969: 66)

If this is true, then people who speak the same language but whose speaking is articulated in a different social universe are best placed to hold up an intelligible mirror to our reality: what is 'natural' to us will be strange to them.

Berger and Luckmann use the term 'reification' for the process whereby human productions come to be understood as independently objective reality. They also point out that the process goes both ways: 'de-reification' can also happen. They even give three examples of 'the social circumstances that favour de-reification': the 'collapse of institutional orders, the contact between previously segregated societies, and the important phenomenon of social marginality' (Berger & Luckmann 1971: 109).

Two of our overseas chapters clearly speak to us from these social conditions; first, 'the contact between previously segregated societies'. O'Brien and Heron relate that

The relationship between the indigenous Maori people and pakeha (non-Maori) New Zealanders, expressed in the 1840 Treaty of Waitangi, is a distinguishing characteristic of New Zealand society. . . . A raft of official documents refers to the need for consultation between the Treaty partners. The Treaty relationship, often expressed as a form of biculturalism[17] . . . underpins all areas of public policy and governance in New Zealand. (Chapter 10.4, pp. 197–98)

Next 'social marginality'. Kathryn Church was de-reifying herself almost before she was reified, preparing herself for her later work at the margins of mainstream Canadian society by attending 'two schools [which were] marginal in different ways within the spectrum of Canadian universities'. The language of de-structuring pervades her account of working as a knowledge producer with psychiatric survivors, especially the paragraphs beginning 'Like a modern-day

---

[17] 'The Treaty relationship, often expressed as a form of bi-culturalism' is an excellent modern example of what Barnes has called a 'social paradigm', in effect a socially embedded belief-and-action system connecting people with shared understandings and expectations of the social world (Barnes 1969). The Recovery movement would be another, which might usefully be compared, as an example of a 'user-led' movement making claims for newly asserted-as-valid identities, with the African self-respect movement of the 1960s called *négritude*. For our purposes here, note especially how, though these are movements of knowledge, they are not contained within the academy: they have moved from esoteric to exoteric.

Penelope . . .' on p. 184 (for relationships themselves) and 'This is an important experience . . .' on p. 183 (for producing knowledge from the experiences). It is surely of the first importance how consistently her account reveals the fragility of structuralism, the ubiquity of marginalisation words: unsettlement, unlearning, differences, outsider, periphery, disembodies, buffers, displaced, doubtful legitimacy/credibility, and more.

However, who writes about 'the collapse of institutional orders'? Answer: all the British. Tilley most explicitly perhaps, and poignantly too, himself in a different sense a 'psychiatric survivor' in what was once a hegemonic institution but is now an influential niche (see Introduction). However, I see all the UK chapters as expressing[18] the shock – through overemphatic resistance to the shock – of the UK's collapse of institutional orders. Church recognises de-reification in the accounts of Chambers *et al.* and Forrest and Masters, as well as in Tilley. Smoyak indirectly diagnoses some such institutional collapse in the – *pace* herself – indignant irritation with which she lists all the things a good institutional account *ought* to have but which these do not. Hazelton picks up Gournay's claim that 'pure mental health nursing research' has died – and therefore (by implication) so too will most of the other authors in the book plus their superseded institutions – as incidentally raising questions over the Australian institutional order as well as the UK's. He catches the political drift in Gournay's institutional description.

Well, what does this amount to? What does reframing through distant lenses allow us to do, beyond opening the door to a recategorisation in sociological terms, to the effect that our authors write as they do because the institutional order within which they are embedded is 'de-reifying'? When the products of the mind become stumbling-blocks, the mind needs to produce new products. An epistemological crisis [which, if indeed it 'is always a crisis in human relationships' (MacIntyre 1989: 243) we have every evidence of having here] is resolved 'by the construction of a new narrative' (MacIntyre 1989: 243). Do our overseas authors confirm this claim? In different ways I believe they do. The Australian attempt to construct a new narrative I have already singled out in an earlier analogy as an attempted metasystem transition, but we can now see it also as an attempt to give authority to a new narrator. Church's chapter is a despatch from the front, reflectively reviewing in first person mode the story of an activist who decided to make her own transition, to begin a shape-shifting narrative of living and working *Like Crazy*: she unilaterally reconstructed her story to align as closely as she (or they) could bear with those of psychiatric survivors. From her social marginality, she realised to some degree the redrafting of the intellectual basis of Canadian mental health institutions that New Zealand seems to have achieved to a nearly complete degree. There the promotion since 1997 of consumer focus and the use of a recovery model as the national policy for mental health amounts to a

---

[18] As would also have expressed, I surmise, the chapters that we do not have, from Barker, Bowers and Brooker.

're-constitution' of the country, an attempt to restart New Zealand history, but this time as the story of a unitary community under a treaty rather than of an indigenous minority under a colonising settler majority. It is noteworthy that O'Brien and Heron, from their more inclusive perspective, see the chapters by Forrest and Masters and Chambers *et al.* more as pleas for rapprochement between the competing traditions than as statements of difference.

Where then does this leave my emphasis on the power of these traditions to form identities as a driver behind the perceived non-dialogue and lack of accommodation to each other's point of view? Is there a new rapprochement narrative underlying these chapters, Schoppman's 'great achievement of integration'? Perhaps – each reader must decide. However, this pressing together of the concepts of (de-)reification and epistemological crisis is intended to push readers to reflect on how they see the circumstances out of which the chapters on nursing knowledge in the UK have come. For myself, I take encouragement from an historical parallel. Alasdair MacIntyre claims that, at a previous transition between major stages of European cultural history, it was the comprehensive genius of Shakespeare that succeeded in portraying how such an era made

> ambiguity, the possibility of alternative interpretations . . . a central feature of human character and activity. *Hamlet* is Shakespeare's brilliant mirror to the age . . . For Shakespeare invites us to reflect upon the crisis of the self as a crisis in the tradition that has formed the self. (MacIntyre 1989: 248)

If sociological fracture is what produces epistemological crisis, epistemological crisis can only be resolved by sociological work. However objectivistic, the human world can be remade by those who made it: the self can make a new tradition. However, to escape the conflict and contradiction we have seen in this book, integrating ideas have to inform comprehensive ('inclusive') institutions. The protracted collapse (evident in the more or less incessant rebuilding) of the 'tradition' of UK public institutions is taking its toll on the identities formed within it. Therefore it is indeed a great achievement of integration that someone (from overseas!) should challenge a sample of stout hearts manning the battlements of that modern Elsinore of ambiguity, the NHS, to essay a collective escape from sociological fracture and epistemological/institutional crisis. Their book may not be the narrative of an integrated policy for mental health in the UK, but it may turn out to be where it started.

References

Barnes, B. (1969) Paradigms – scientific and social. *Man* New Series, 4 (1): 94–102.
Ben-David, J. & Collins, R. (1966) Social factors in the origins of a new science: the case of psychology. *American Sociological Review*, 31 (4): 451–65.
Berger, P.L. & Luckmann, T. (1969) Sociology of religion and sociology of knowledge. In: *Sociology of Religion: Selected Readings* (ed. R. Robertson). Harmondsworth: Penguin, pp. 61–73.

Berger, P.L. & Luckmann, T. (1971) *The Social Construction of Reality: A Treatise in the Sociology of Knowledge.* Harmondsworth: Penguin.

Bowers, L. (1992) Ethnomethodology II: a study of the Community Psychiatric Nurse in the patient's home. *International Journal of Nursing Studies*, 29 (1): 69–79.

Bucher, R. & Strauss, A. (1961) Professions in process. *American Journal of Sociology*, 66: 325–34.

Clark, D.H. (1964) *Administrative Therapy: The Role of the Doctor in the Therapeutic Community.* London: Tavistock.

Corney, R.H. (1996) Links between mental health care professionals and general practices in England and Wales: the impact of GP fundholding. *British Journal of General Practice*, 46: 221–4.

Deegan, P. (1996) Recovery as a journey of the heart. *Psychiatric Rehabilitation Journal*, 19 (3): 91–7.

Glaser, B.G. & Strauss, A.L. (1967) *The Discovery of Grounded Theory: Strategies for Qualitative Research.* Chicago: Aldine.

Gournay, K. & Brooking, J. (1993) Failure and dissatisfaction. In: *Community Psychiatric Nursing: A Research Perspective, Volume 2* (eds C. Brooker & E. White). London: Chapman and Hall.

James, W. (1907) *Talks to Teachers on Psychology: and to Students on Some of Life's Ideals* Longman, Green & Co, London.

Kuhn, T.S. (1970) *The Structure of Scientific Revolutions*, enlarged edn. Chicago: Chicago University Press.

Lave, J. (1986) The values of quantification. In: *Power, Action and Belief: A New Sociology of Knowledge?* (ed. J. Law), pp. 88–111. London: Routledge and Kegan Paul.

MacIntyre, A. (1989) Epistemological crises, dramatic narrative and the philosophy of science. In: *Anti-theory in Ethics and Moral Conservatism* (eds S.G. Clarke & E. Simpson), pp. 241–61. Albany: SUNY Press.

Parkin, F. (1982) *Max Weber.* Chichester/London: Ellis Horwood/Tavistock.

Polanyi, M. & Prosch, H. (1975) *Meaning.* Chicago: Chicago University Press.

Prior, L. (1993) *The Social Organization of Mental Illness.* London: Sage.

Rapaport, R.N. (1960) *Community as Doctor: New Perspectives on a Therapeutic Community.* London: Tavistock.

Roosens, E. (1979) *Mental Patients in Town Life: Geel – Europe's First Therapeutic Community.* London: Sage.

Ryan, D. (1997) Ambiguity in nursing: the person and the organisation as contrasting sources of meaning in nursing practice. In: *The Mental Health Nurse: Views of Practice and Education* (ed. S. Tilley), pp. 118–36. Oxford: Blackwell Science.

Ryan, D., Tilley, S. & Pollock, L. (1998) *Review of Literature on the Effectiveness of Community Psychiatric Nurses in Achieving Health Outcomes for People with Mental Illness. Report to the Chief Scientist Office, Department of Health, Scottish Office.* Edinburgh: Department of Nursing Studies, University of Edinburgh.

Samson, C. (1995) The fracturing of medical dominance in British psychiatry?, *Sociology of Health and Illness*, 17 (2): 245–68.

Schneider, D.M. (1976) Notes toward a theory of culture. In: *Meaning in Anthropology* (eds K.H. Basso & H.A. Selby), pp. 197–200. Albuquerque: University of New Mexico Press.

Shepherd, M. (1993) Foreword, In: *Integrated Mental Health Care* (eds I.R.H. Falloon & G. Fadden). Cambridge: Cambridge University Press.

Shepherd, M., Murray, A. & Muijen, M. (1995) Perspectives on schizophrenia: a survey of user, family carer and professional views regarding effective care. *Journal of Mental Health*, 4,: 403–22.

Szasz, T.S. (1966) The mental health ethic. In: *Ethics and Society: Original Essays on Contemporary Moral Problems* (ed. R.T. De George), pp. 85–110. Garden City, New York: Doubleday Anchor.

Turchin, V. (1981) *The Inertia of Fear and the Scientific Worldview* (translated by G. Daniels). Oxford: Martin Robertson.

Wigglesworth, V.B. (1968) *The Life of Insects.* New York: Mentor Books.

Chapter 12

Conclusion: From the Towers to the Piazza

Stephen Tilley

This book was intended as a study of the field of knowledge in psychiatric and mental health nursing, with particular reference to its institutionalisation in UK higher education. In asking my fellow UK authors to discuss the knowledge that they saw as dominant in their own institutions, my intentions were to set in motion a collaborative inquiry and to achieve a collective view. The collaborative inquiry was to be structured by the process of mutual reading of and commenting on texts; the collective view was to be facilitated by the use of the objectifying matrix constructed, with Ryan's help, in the Introduction. To what extent has the original aim of the book been achieved? Equally importantly, what unexpected findings have we made, and what productive insights gained?

The most immediate finding is that the best-laid plans of mice and book editors 'gang aft agly'. First, authors were scrupulous in reading each others' texts, but the resultant discussion seems not to have come out as fully collaborative as I intended. Second, the would-be facilitating matrix was obviously not experienced as such, since there was scarcely any reference to it in any chapter. Third, the reader will have found some authors questioning whether *the* field, or even *a* field, has been identified clearly or adequately. In this concluding chapter I would like to address these apparent shortfalls from the originating design, to read them for what they do nevertheless tell us about the field of psychiatric and mental health nursing knowledge.

I will begin with the question of the degree to which the discussion of each others' chapters was collaborative. The more external commentators thought they could identify a breakdown in relationships in the knowledge communities relevant to mental health, visible in the incomplete mutual recognition by the authors, and their failure to engage in dialogue. These issues were addressed most specifically in Chapter 11, where Ryan suggested a possible reason for the communication deficit in the existence of unresolved tensions at higher levels of the mental health system, a consequence of the piecemeal change imposed on the system over the last 20 years. These unresolved tensions leave knowledge specialists in a contradictory position, caught in an 'epistemological crisis' between the claims of scientific knowledge (validated methodologically) and the claims of service users/survivors (whose knowledge is validated experientially). This sociological reframing of the dialogic process of the book helps me to see that the original aspiration that authors should work 'collaboratively' was more a product of how I then saw the field than how it has turned out to be. I presumed the field of knowledge was more self-contained than in fact it is, and that academics were more autonomous than in fact we are. Powerful external forces run through the field, destabilising both the forms of usable knowledge and the relations among knowledge users. Hence the book is itself a symptom of the fragility of the boundaries delineating the field. This is an unexpected finding of some importance.

Next, why was there so little use of the matrix? While it is true that the authors of Chapters 2–8 were not constrained to use it, they were *offered* a model within which to situate their reflections. The model identified four forms of institutionalisation of knowledge, in an ascending rank of social power: influence, tradition, discipline and institution. Their putative connections in a dynamic sequence were presented in the novel form of a spiral four-cell table. While I am happy to say that the book we have is more interesting than the book I planned, it is nonetheless fruitful to see how some chapters can be placed on the spiral. Readers may have been doing so already, in which case similarities and differences between their maps and mine will be data in an as yet undocumented extension of the process of this book.

Recalling the working definition of *institutions* as 'politico-economic structures which publicly hold knowledge which is interest-bearing, consensually validated, usable . . . taken from disciplines and traditions . . . filtered through a mesh of political judgements as to practicability, congruence with political interests, etc.' (Chapter 1), we must see Gournay's knowledge claims as most institutionally authoritative. By comparison with Griffiths and Franks' account of the Tavistock–Cassel-Middlesex nexus, he shows how success at the level of the institution both feeds off and reacts back on practices at the level of the *discipline*. The forms of knowledge are disciplinary matters, yet they have impact on the institution (e.g. in attracting funding, students, attention from policy makers), as does the institution have impact on the discipline (e.g. neither psychodynamic knowledge nor cognitive-behavioural psychology are unreservedly accepted approaches in mental health care). Tilley's University of Edinburgh mental health nursing knowledge could be seen as borderline *tradition*: its paradigmatic form of knowledge is the values-based doctoral study critiquing practice. Norman's account of knowledge at King's College (according to his commentary in Chapter 9.7) likewise has some characteristics of both discipline and school/tradition. Carson, in his exemplarily critical self-reflection, most clearly acts at the level of *influence*, the 'individual scholar in his garret' helping colleagues to see 'a better version of themselves' [Weaver, cited in Szasz (1979: 20)]. However, the psychiatric services users – who we now acknowledge as co-constructors of this field of knowledge – are also unable to rise above the level of influence. Through involvement with users, Forrest and Masters influence educational practice in the form of curriculum, but apparently influence only some of their colleagues to become collaborators in the process. Chambers *et al.*'s chapter conveys a sense of the authors being influenced by their own experiences of living and working across the user/provider fault line, and of influencing each other in writing their chapter.

Use of the matrix indicates some anomalies or ironies. On the one hand, if we see Gournay's institution 'seeking to impose a practice – based on "science"',, we also see that it does not fully 'control practice', at least some other authors' knowledge-producing practice ('more ad hoc, occasioned, circumstantial, "art"'). The UK knowledge system is still highly pluralistic. Nonetheless, its ubiquitous appearance as reference point underscores the power of Gournay's institution. This institutional power, however, is not pure disciplinary (and therefore professional) power: as Ryan notes in Chapter 11, at the Institute, at both institutional and disciplinary level, nursing is part of a psychiatry-led multidisciplinary whole. We see this permeability of nursing knowledge at the discipline level elsewhere: for the Tavistock/Cassel, King's College and the University of Edinburgh, the prevalent paradigms are those of other disciplines. The key to influence, we might say, is the 'personal permeability' of the 'targeted agent'. Kathryn Church, Forrest and Masters and Chambers *et al.* are the most powerful examples of influence: influence by users, or mutual influence by the authors, or by one's own experience. In all cases engagement with users' lifeworld and experiential knowledge unsettles the professionals' knowledge base. Once again, disciplinary knowledge and user experience come into tension.

The matrix had as one dimension theoretical/practical, as the other personal/ political. Arranging the authors of Chapters 2–9 on this grid gives hardly any undistributed placings (perhaps only Carson in the personal/practical cell), thereby stimulating some interesting questions. So Forrest and Masters would seem to be primarily located in the personal/practical quadrant although, as their research was funded and disseminated by the Scottish national nursing body, disciplinary aspects are evident too. Griffiths and Franks seem clearly to fit the personal/theoretical quadrant, while also intersecting the practical/political, with accounts of English national recognition and funding of psychodynamic courses. Where does this place psychodynamic knowledge in terms of its standing as an academic discipline? While Gournay is clearly in the political/practical quadrant, there are clear threads through the discipline, the school and personal influence quadrant (e.g. his highlighting of David Goldberg's influence as mentor). This suggests that the model points to the cumulative rather than substitutive nature of the spiraling progress through the quadrants. Does effective knowledge as power have four levels? Is it a multi-level integration rather than a top-level emergence?

Using the matrix as above supplements the observations made by international commentators that either the chapters fall into two clusters with variations (e.g. those focused on the nurse–patient relationship and those focused on therapy or management of illness) or a continuum of paradigms can be discerned. So far, so static. Activating the matrix allows us to see the constructions of knowledge in institutions as reflecting political ambitions and rhetorical intent, i.e. as dynamic, not static. Mapping the matrix analysis onto others' analyses, we notice that those 'lower' on the spiral are indeed most closely involved with users in relationships of knowledge production which 'unsettle' their relationships with academic colleagues and the higher education institutions [Bannerji, quoted in

Church (1995)]. This is the case, in different ways, and with degrees of 'unsettle-ment', for Chambers *et al.*, Forrest and Masters, and Carson.[1]

Where, through engagement with users, the political system changes in va-lence towards a micro-politics of meaning (cf. Doyle McCarthy 1996), knowledge in institutions becomes an open frontier. Perhaps here we begin to reach from matrix to metaphor. The field is to some degree a 'frontier': it is less than fully regulated; identities and the power to determine what 'counts as knowledge' are open to negotiation and competition. However, it is also to some degree 'settled' territory, macro-politically ruled, with local power-holders institutionalising their accepted resources of knowledge in well-defended towers. It is the cultural shift towards a micro-politics of meaning within the field of services in general that shows up these political towers as signs of breakdown of relationship in the macro-politically ruled knowledge community. To extend the claim made above, micropolitical engagement with users' lifeworlds and experiential knowledge unsettles the professionals' relationship with their field of knowledge, in particu-lar the disciplinary and institutional quadrants of the matrix.

This would be consistent with variation in use of the term 'field' in Chapters 2–8 and commentaries in Chapter 9, where some writers see themselves as working in a corner of the field, others in a field among fields. The coordinating status of 'the field' concept was not assured. Since the primary object of concern of the book has come to be questioned rather than taken for granted, it is not surprising that no use was made of the situating scheme from the Introduction. As we have just seen, it can still be pressed into useful service, and some insights of a broad sociological kind have emerged. However, the neglect of the model and the lack of confidence that there actually *is* such a thing as a field of PMHNing know-ledge make a conventional revisiting of the issues presented in the Introduction problematic: it would not be doing justice to what has been written. We have no option therefore, but to go back even further, to return to the metaphors that helped in the conception of the book and to consider what light they shed on how the book has actually turned out.

The conversation, the tower and the piazza

First, the conversation. I ended *The Mental Health Nurse* (Tilley 1997) with an image of the square at Duns, seeing it as a metaphor for centuries of rhetorical arguments over interpretations of texts: what version would be accepted as the basis for deciding how personal, moral, political life was to go on? In the square at Duns, one man spoke, everyone else listened (bar qualifying asides which were not intended to engage the speaker in dialogue). This picture of a monopolistic

---

[1] The matrix could likewise be used to analyse commentaries by international contributors – particu-larly their comparative comments on discipline and institution.

commitment to a single conduct-determining text was taken as an anti-model: I concluded that there neither could nor ought to be a single authoritative text for mental health nursing. Contesting versions of texts (about PMHNing) is vital in constructing a pluralistic community of practice and education, and readers must judge each author's/speaker's appeal to determine to what and to whom to respond.

In this book some overseas commentators noted a lack of dialogue among the UK institutional authors. It is perhaps worth saying that I was less aware of this absence than they were; what they saw as absence of dialogue I felt might instead be negotiating/seeking/setting the terms for dialogue – each chapter's author(s) trying to hold onto their own truth, to preserve their integrity and individuality. Each is saying not just 'this variety of practice (of knowledge production) is worth preserving' but 'I/we am/are worth preserving'. Some kind of conversation there was, however – though perhaps rather interior, even virtual. One contributor from Section 1, Carson, said he had enjoyed reading all the commentaries by other authors in that section and that it would be good to have another 'round' of that. Furthermore, Schoppmann, an international commentator who noted an absence of dialogue, said that she had carried on 'lots of imagined conversations with each one (of the UK authors)'.[2] Some form of dialogue (including imaginary) seems to extend beyond these pages; inward, in the minds of the contributors, and outward, as desired extension of the project.

Our metaphors are running us into difficulties. Turning first to the tower: this was a metaphor that explicitly guided the production of accounts of knowledge, since authors were asked to envisage themselves as looking out from the tower of their institution and asked to describe what they saw. The tower that imaginatively underlay this task was not much more sophisticated than an elevated platform, a vantage point for reflexive observation of one's own locus of knowledge production, and for straightforward observation of others; a kind of lighthouse with an eye instead of a beacon. However, not all towers are like this. By chance, not a mile away from where I work there is a tower of a very different sort, one that was originally conceived with a deep historical and philosophical purpose: the Outlook Tower of Patrick Geddes. In Edinburgh, an old volcanic spine runs eastward from the castle to Arthur's Seat. Adjacent to the castle is a tower which, since the 1850s, has housed a *camera obscura* (Latin for 'dark chamber' or 'dark room'). The *camera obscura* consists of a periscope extended above the top of the tower, through which light enters to be reflected by a mirror onto a concave, white-painted circular table top in a darkened room. Images of the

---

[2] 'I was not very satisfied with the further commentaries. For me the aim of the whole book seems to be the integration of different view points in psychiatric nursing and I was hoping that the authors, after reading the others' contributions, would try to come into a dialogue together; but in my view this did not really happen. Instead I found that everyone took the chance to clarify their own position again . . . I can tell you that I had lots of imagined conversations which each of them.' (Susanne Schoppmann, personal communication)

prospects visible from the tower are thus transposed inside, in miniature. By operating two controls one can focus on different aspects of the view, zooming in or out.

What has this to do with the matters of concern in this book? In the 1890s Patrick Geddes visited the *camera obscura* and immediately saw 'the Outlook Tower as a way to resolve what he saw as an "evolutionary crisis"' – a 'three-fold breakdown between individuals and their spatial, temporal and cultural environment' (Chabard 2004). For Geddes, the tower offered a means of 're-situating the individual in the world[,] the basic condition for changing the course of human evolution and opening up a brighter future'. Geddes emphasised the 'fundamental importance of vision in the organisation and orchestration of the Tower', and in its role in resolving

> a breakdown between the individual and his environment. By re-articulating the landscape and its history, he aimed to re-situate visitors in the evolutionary cycle by helping them to become citizens capable of envisaging and building their own future and, collectively, that of their city. (Chabard 2004)

The reader may now begin to see parallels between Geddes' project and ours in this book. The counterpart breakdown in our account of the field of knowledge of PMHNing is the breakdown between individuals (nurses and users) and their institutional spatial (community and hospital), temporal (hospital-based to higher education-based) and cultural (social production and consumption of knowledge about mental health) environment. In all of these spheres what is missing is the capacity to transcend the institutions that create knowledge. What is needed is something that would 'break down' the breakdown.

In Chapter 11, Ryan diagnosed an unresolved social fracture and evolutionary crisis:

> In view of the contradictory coexistence of residential hospitals and community care, it is reasonable to describe the field within which nursing has to make its way as a metathetelic monster (Wigglesworth 1968: 111), functionally enlarged but not morphologically developed, frozen in mid-metamorphosis with characteristics of both 'stages'. (Ryan, Chapter 11, p. 226)

His 'relativising' analysis, like Geddes', brings into focus 'hidden' dimensions of the environment – spatial (hospital to community; the international contributors distanced from, but now 'visible' to, the UK); temporal (UK contributors' references to the asylum past; overseas to their histories); and cultural (cultural contexts made relevant by UK and overseas contributors). His analytical ascent is brother to Geddes' climb up (and down) the Outlook Tower; the epistemological crisis he draws from MacIntyre is akin to the breakdown between individuals and their cultural environment, diagnosed by Geddes as precipitating a crisis of urban civilisation, of the city.

The visual metaphor was much used by those involved in the 'care wars'; the 'proper focus' of PMHNing was a subject of heated debate (e.g. Barker & Reynolds 1996; Repper, 2000). However, there is vision and vision: a seeing of the biological eye, and a seeing of the inner eye, the spiritual eye. Geddes was indeed preoccupied with looking out, with panoramas and outlooks, with landscapes and cityscapes; but these were instrumental: his ultimate quarry was the kind of epistemological shift Ryan attributes to Galileo, an irreversible alteration in the way we understand, not just a new take on what we see. By 're-locating' his visitors into a new articulation of landscape and history, he intended them to be transformed into 'citizens', active members of a civilisation, living stones 'building their own future and, collectively, that of their city'.

We need therefore to go beyond 'tower' and 'conversation'. Our authors challenge us to go beyond both my hope that a plurivocal conversation might supplant the would-be hegemonic monologue in the square at Duns and Ryan's hope that the self might make a new tradition. We need to take on Geddes' larger vision of a civilisation, a dynamic ensemble of many traditions sharing a determinate space and collectively constructing the wellbeing of each and of all. What is needed is a change of vision; not of the field alone, of prospect or aspect, but of vision itself.[3] We therefore need to undertake an epistemological shift with our metaphors, our 'think-withs' (Hodgkin 1997). The tower *from which* we observe the field must give way to the tower *within which* we (seek to) change our outlook. We must undertake 'new forms of interaction between [ourselves] and the surrounding world, institute interaction between [ourselves] based on thought' (Chabard 2004)[4]. For Geddes himself the visionary civilisation that would be the achievement of new forms of interaction was instantiated in his 'University Hall scheme'. He intended to transform the Old Town slum in which the Outlook Tower stood 'into an Edinburgh "Latin Quarter", based on the model of the medieval University or "Cloister". Complete with students, refectories . . . all run by the students themselves in a spirit of brotherly freedom'. The Outlook Tower, in short, 'was gradually being absorbed into Geddes's [larger] scheme', the renovation or 'cultural rehabilitation' which Geddes saw as 'achievable only if the historic city . . . becomes recognised as the place to achieve any improvement in the city' (Welter, cited in Chabard, 2004). He never secured the authority to effect a similar transformation in Edinburgh. However, he did build – and right beside the Outlook Tower – the germ of his visionary civilisation in the form of a multifunction, democratically run University Hall, 'the first conceptual context for the Outlook Tower' (Chabard 2004).

---

[3] 'Nature centers into balls
   And her proud ephemerals,
   Fast to surface and outside
   Scan the surface of the sphere.
   Knew they what that signified
   New genesis were here.' (Emerson 1841)
[4] The eye is the 'optic chiasma' conjoining the view outward and the view inward (Chabard 2004).

Geddes' Outlook Tower, therefore, is only half the picture. What you saw when you looked out from the tower of the outer eye was the tower of the inner eye: the aspect gave on to the vision.[5] This vision was a form of urban healing, for his reaction to the civic and urban dysfunction of 'paleotechnic' industrialism was to seek

> to restore the lost relationship between individuals and their urban and geographical space, their historic heritage and the universal body of knowledge accumulated by men. (Chabard 2004)[6]

We are back with knowledge. Universal, not institutional. Our detour through metaphor brings us up against a vision of wholeness, but we also fall in with an optimism about history and a trust in intelligence at what was a very confused moment in the understanding of post-industrial urbanism. In the chapter by O'Brien and Heron we come closest to what one might call 'Geddesian conversion experience', a paradigm shift from the functional improvement of service delivery systems to the inauguration of a new civilisation: 'the Treaty relationship'. Mental health in New Zealand is part of a vision of a society, a civilisation to be aspired after for all citizens, to be built by the citizens.[7] Such a society does not promote the kind of defensive/aggressive towers that bring discord and division to the city; rather it seeks to bring the leaders into the council chamber and the citizenry into the piazza: from discord to discussion, from monologue to dialogue.

Geddes' visionary University Hall project is in effect a North Italian city piazza[8] folded in on itself: it has the potential to perform the functions to regenerate a civilisation, but without open access and not in the open air. It is a site for discoursing, but in a more engaged (it is 'democratically run', and therefore civilising) way than that found in the square at Duns: where rhetoric is met not with tolerant silence but instead collective counter-rhetoric. Here is seen a culture that constructs speakers who can listen, forms of knowledge that universalise and, at the same time, institutions that can respond.[9]

---

[5] The vision was actively constructed. Geddes asked people to run up the five flights of stairs to the rampart, then re-enter and view the camera obscura, before descending successive floors in which one encountered diverse scientific and other instruments, metonymically focusing both outward and inward eye on a new sense of vision. (Cf. The diverse forms in which authors displayed their intra- and inter-tower observations.)

[6] This appeal to universal (and 'men's') knowledge may jar with ours to local, disputed knowledges.

[7] See, for example, the definition of 'recovery' at the heart of New Zealand's mental health strategy: 'the ability to live well in the presence or absence of mental illness (or whatever the person chooses to name it).' (Mental Health Commission 2001: 1)

[9] Another example of an unfolded piazza is the Raging Spoon Café in Toronto, exemplar in the National Film Board of Canada documentary *Working Like Crazy* (Basen & Sky, 1999), of survivor-run businesses and community economic development.

Working from this comparison, I believe this book has amply delivered on the expectations appropriate to the first tower, the Outlook Tower: so much so that we, all the authors of the chapters and all the colleagues we speak for, now have the resources to converge on the second tower, to 'go down to the piazza' and take history forward. We now see that the astonishing diversity in these texts is not a difficulty but a strength – our professional civilisation has so many traditions, and these are so well spoken for. We now see that our authors are just as sensitive as Geddes to the dysfunctional impact of undigested change on people's capacity to maintain their mental wellbeing and the relationships that underpin it.

There are many indicators of sensitivity to that impact, and signs that capacity can be maintained and change digested. I will note six that have resonated particularly with me. The first is Church sensitising us to the role that *personal and institutional history* ('where we've been'[10]) plays in determining how we answer the questions 'Who is this field of knowledge for?' and 'Whose interests does it serve?'. The second is sensitivity to issues of thinking and writing across *differences*, enabling negotiation of 'indigestible' change, e.g. in the process of work in Chambers *et al.*'s chapter and in Forrest and Masters' work on user involvement. The third is the sensitivity displayed by several of the authors in rising from the level of practice and curriculum to that of the *principles and values* that should guide those endeavours. The fourth is shown by the convergence of emphasis – across even apparent 'binary divides' – on *relationship* as key to the development of knowledge in the field. The fifth is the sensitivity shown by the authors in this collaborative enquiry, working across disciplinary, institutional, existential and cultural boundaries and in richly varied languages, to what is involved in trying to imagine and construct a *'balanced knowledge base'*[11]. The sixth sensitivity I discern in signs of spirited commitment to (personal, professional and institutional) *recovery*: our collective 'ability to live well in the presence or absence of one's mental illness (or whatever people choose to name their experience)' (Mental Health Commission 2001: 1).

The diversity of traditions shown here does not inevitably incite an epistemological crisis, nor is the UK mental health system forever doomed not to digest change. However, institutions have the power in the modern world, as Geddes realised early on. In order to transcend monologue and defensiveness, one creates institutions for dialogue and open inclusiveness.

---

[10] This is taken from the title of Kathryn Church's text on survivor-run businesses in Toronto: *Because of Where We've Been: The Business Behind the Business of Psychiatric Survivor Economic Development* (Church 1997).

[11] The *New Framework for Support* (Trainor *et al.* 1993) posits a 'balanced' 'knowledge resource base' comprising medical/clinical, social science, experiential, and customary/traditional knowledge as a key requisite for shifting to and supporting a 'community resource' approach to mental health services.

References

Barker, P.J. & Reynolds, B. (1996) Rediscovering the proper focus of nursing: a critique of Gournay's position on nursing theory and models. *Journal of Psychiatric and Mental Health Nursing*, 3 (1): 76–80.

Basen, G. & Sky, L. (1999) *Working Like Carzy* [documentary film]. Montreal, PQ: National Film Board of Canada and Sky Works Charitable Foundation.

Chabard, P. (2004) *The Outlook Tower as an Anamorphosis of the World: Patrick Geddes and the Theme of Vision*. English translation by Charlotte Ellis. http://www.hodgers.com/mike/patrickgeddes/feature_eleven.html

Church, K. (1995) *Forbidden Narratives: Critical Autobiography as Social Science*. Gordon & Breach: Luxembourg.

Church, K. (1997) *Because of Where We've Been: The Business Behind the Business of Psychiatric Survivor Economic Development*. Toronto: Ontario Council of Alternative Businesses in Partnership with 761 Community Development Corporation.

Doyle McCarthy, E. (1996) *Knowledge as Culture: The New Sociology of Knowledge*. London: Routledge.

Emerson, R.W. (1841) Circles. In: *Emerson (1982) Selected Essays* (edited and with an introduction by L. Ziff), pp. 225–38. Harmondsworth: Penguin.

Hodgkin, R.A. (1997) Making space for meaning. *Oxford Review of Education*, 23 (3): 385–99.

Mental Health Commission (2001) *Recovery Competencies for New Zealand Mental Health Workers*. Wellington: MHC.

Repper, J. (2000) Adjusting the focus of mental health nursing: incorporating service users' experiences of recovery. *Journal of Mental Health*, 9 (6): 575–88.

Szasz, T. (1979) *The Myth of Psychotherapy: Mental Healing as Religion, Rhetoric and Repression*. Oxford: Oxford University Press.

Tilley, S. (ed.) (1997) *The Mental Health Nurse: Views of Practice and Education*. Oxford: Blackwell Science.

Trainor, J., Pomeroy, E. & Pape, B. (1993) A new framework for support (edited and abridged). In: *Building a Framework for Support* (eds J. Trainor, E. Pomeroy & B. Pape). Toronto: Canadian Mental Health Association.

Index

Page numbers in italics refer to figures or tables.